Food Labels

Recent Titles in
Q&A Health Guides

FOOD LABELS

Your Questions Answered

Barbara A. Brehm

Q&A Health Guides

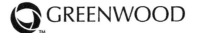

GREENWOOD

An Imprint of ABC-CLIO, LLC
Santa Barbara, California • Denver, Colorado

Library of Congress Cataloging in Publication Control Number: 2019033120

ISBN: 978-1-4408-6366-0 (print)
       978-1-4408-6367-7 (ebook)

23 22 21 20 19   1 2 3 4 5

This book is also available as an eBook.

Greenwood
An Imprint of ABC-CLIO, LLC

ABC-CLIO, LLC
147 Castilian Drive
Santa Barbara, California 93117
www.abc-clio.com

This book is printed on acid-free paper ∞

Manufactured in the United States of America

This book discusses treatments (including types of medication and mental health therapies), diagnostic tests for various symptoms and mental health disorders, and organizations. The author has made every effort to present accurate and up-to-date information. However, the information in this book is not intended to recommend or endorse particular treatments or organizations, or substitute for the care or medical advice of a qualified health professional, or used to alter any medical therapy without a medical doctor's advice. Specific situations may require specific therapeutic approaches not included in this book. For those reasons, we recommend that readers follow the advice of qualified health care professionals directly involved in their care. Readers who suspect they may have specific medical problems should consult a physician about any suggestions made in this book.

Contents

Series Foreword

All of us have questions about our health. Is this normal? Should I be doing something differently? Whom should I talk to about my concerns? And our modern world is full of answers. Thanks to the Internet, there's a wealth of information at our fingertips, from forums where people can share their personal experiences to Wikipedia articles to the full text of medical studies. But finding the right information can be an intimidating and difficult task—some sources are written at too high a level, others have been oversimplified, while still others are heavily biased or simply inaccurate.

Q&A Health Guides address the needs of readers who want accurate, concise answers to their health questions, authored by reputable and objective experts, and written in clear and easy-to-understand language. This series focuses on the topics that matter most to young adult readers, including various aspects of physical and emotional well-being as well as other components of a healthy lifestyle. These guides will also serve as a valuable tool for parents, school counselors, and others who may need to answer teens' health questions.

All books in the series follow the same format to make finding information quick and easy. Each volume begins with an essay on health literacy and why it is so important when it comes to gathering and evaluating health information. Next, the top five myths and misconceptions that surround the topic are dispelled. The heart of each guide is a collection of questions and answers, organized thematically. A selection of five case studies provides real-world examples to illuminate key concepts. Rounding out each volume are a directory of resources, glossary, and index.

It is our hope that the books in this series will not only provide valuable information but will also help guide readers toward a lifetime of healthy decision making.

Acknowledgments

I would like to acknowledge with heartfelt gratitude my colleagues in the Department of Exercise and Sport Studies at Smith College, especially Lynn Oberbillig who took over all chair responsibilities during my sabbatical semester and always does more than her share of the heavy lifting in administrative work for our department. Sarah Witkowski has steadily helped steer our ship in productive directions so that I was able to give more thought to this project. Our administrative assistant Rachel Cook always keeps the ball rolling no matter what difficulties arise. We are a good team!

Many thanks to Smith College for the support of my sabbatical leave, and for the many ways Smith supports faculty development at all stages of our careers. Thanks also to my nutrition and my sports nutrition students who ask interesting questions and help keep me in touch with the issues important to young people today. My student advisees in Smith's Sustainable Food Concentration at Smith have been especially inspirational to work with.

Thanks also to my family and friends who shared their questions about food labels and gave feedback on essays. Thanks especially to my sons Ian, for sharing a writers' retreat with me, and Adam, for conversations about food, for his concern for environmental sustainability, and making me drink a smoothie with dried crickets in it.

Thanks to all farmers raising food, including those in my family, the hill towns of Western Massachusetts, and farmers around the world. I am also grateful to the local groups I have gotten to know that educate young people about growing food, especially the Hartsbrook Waldorf School and Hampshire College.

And finally, many thanks to Maxine Taylor at Greenwood/ABC-CLIO for her ideas and support throughout this project. This book was her inspiration, and I have thoroughly enjoyed working on it. Thanks also to Michelle Scott and the team at Greenwood that turned my manuscript into a book.

Introduction

Food labels provide a lot of helpful information to people who take the time to read them. The purpose of this book is to answer questions people have about the information they find on food labels. While much of this information is fairly straightforward, it makes more sense when consumers have a context for understanding what all the text and numbers really mean.

Because food label information is condensed, and must fit into a small area—the food label—it must be general; not all of the information, especially nutrient values, applies to each consumer. In addition, the packaging on food products is a combination of advertising and regulated claims. It is important for consumers to know which is which, and what the regulated claims actually mean.

This book opens with the most common misconceptions many people hold about the information on food labels, then specifically answers important questions about the regulation and meaning of information found on food labels. The first section addresses the regulation of food labels (How are food labels regulated in the United States?) and questions about label accuracy (How accurate is the information on food labels?). The next section dives into questions about the information on the Nutrition Facts panel (What are Daily Values, and what does % Daily Value mean?). Many people rely on food labels to avoid certain ingredients, especially allergens. A section on using the ingredient list and allergen statement helps consumers with important, even life-saving, questions in this area. The last set of questions looks at other labels and claims found on food labels, exploring questions about health claims (What health claims are allowed on food labels, and who decides whether a product label can include that claim?), along with questions about non-GMO, organic, and humane treatment of animal certifications. The book concludes with examples of people using the information on food labels in a variety of ways, a glossary of relevant terms, and a list of resources that may be helpful to readers.

Developing healthy eating habits helps to prevent the chronic diseases that are the leading causes of death and disability in North America and around the world. For healthy living, knowledge is power. Food labels address the belief of many people that personal choice is important for their own health; for the health of family members for whom they prepare food; and for the health of farmers, food producers, and the environment. I hope that by better understanding the information provided by food labels, readers will use that power to make healthful choices, for themselves and for the world.

Guide to Health Literacy

In her 13th year, Samantha was diagnosed with type 2 diabetes. She consulted her mom and her aunt, both of whom also have type 2 diabetes, and decided to go with their strategy of managing diabetes by taking insulin. As a result of participating in an after-school program at her middle school that focused on health literacy, she learned that she can help manage the level of glucose in her bloodstream by counting her carbohydrate intake, following a diabetic diet, and exercising regularly. But, what exactly should she do? How does she keep track of her carbohydrate intake? What is a diabetic diet? How long should she exercise, and what type of exercise should she do? Samantha is a visual learner, so she turned to her favorite source of media, YouTube, to answer these questions. She found videos from individuals around the world sharing their experiences and tips, doctors (or at least people who have "Dr." in their YouTube channel names), government agencies such as the National Institutes of Health, and even video clips from cat lovers who have cats with diabetes. With guidance from the librarian and the health and science teachers at her school, she assessed the credibility of the information in these videos and even compared their suggestions to some of the print resources that she was able to find at her school library. Now, she knows exactly how to count her carbohydrate level, how to prepare and follow a diabetic diet, and how much (and what) exercise is needed daily. She intends to share her findings with her mom and her aunt, and now she wants to create a chart that summarizes what she has learned that she can share with her doctor.

Samantha's experience is not unique. She represents a shift in our society; an individual no longer views himself or herself as a passive recipient of medical care but as an active mediator of his or her own health. However, in this era when any individual can post his or her opinions and experiences with a particular health condition online with just a few clicks or publish a memoir, it is vital that people know how to assess the credibility of health information. Gone are the days when "publishing" health information required intense vetting. The health information landscape is highly saturated, and people have innumerable sources where they can find information about practically any health topic. The sources (whether print, online, or a person) that an individual consults for health information are crucial because the accuracy and trustworthiness of the information can potentially affect his or her overall health. The ability to find, select, assess, and use health information constitutes a type of literacy—health literacy—that everyone must possess.

THE DEFINITION AND PHASES OF HEALTH LITERACY

One of the most popular definitions for health literacy comes from Ratzan and Parker (2000), who describe health literacy as "the degree to which individuals have the capacity to obtain, process, and understand basic health information and services needed to make appropriate health decisions." Recent research has extrapolated health literacy into health literacy bits, further shedding light on the multiple phases and literacy practices that are embedded within the multifaceted concept of health literacy. Although this research has focused primarily on online health information seeking, these health literacy bits are needed to successfully navigate both print and online sources. There are six phases of health information seeking: (1) Information Need Identification and Question Formulation, (2) Information Search, (3) Information Comprehension, (4) Information Assessment, (5) Information Management, and (6) Information Use.

The first phase is the *information need identification and question formulation phase*. In this phase, one needs to be able to develop and refine a range of questions to frame one's search and understand relevant health terms. In the second phase, *information search*, one has to possess appropriate searching skills, such as using proper keywords and correct spelling in search terms, especially when using search engines and databases.

It is also crucial to understand how search engines work (i.e., how search results are derived, what the order of the search results means, how to use the snippets that are provided in the search results list to select websites, and how to determine which listings are ads on a search engine results page). One also has to limit reliance on surface characteristics, such as the design of a website or a book (a website or book that appears to have a lot of information or looks aesthetically pleasant does not necessarily mean it has good information) and language used (a website or book that utilizes jargon, the keywords that one used to conduct the search, or the word "information" does not necessarily indicate it will have good information). The next phase is *information comprehension*, whereby one needs to have the ability to read, comprehend, and recall the information (including textual, numerical, and visual content) one has located from the books and/or online resources.

To assess the credibility of health information (*information assessment* phase), one needs to be able to evaluate information for accuracy, evaluate how current the information is (e.g., when a website was last updated or when a book was published), and evaluate the creators of the source—for example, examine site sponsors or type of sites (.com, .gov, .edu, or .org) or the author of a book (practicing doctor, a celebrity doctor, a patient of a specific disease, etc.) to determine the believability of the person/organization providing the information. Such credibility perceptions tend to become generalized, so they must be frequently reexamined (e.g., the belief that a specific news agency always has credible health information needs continuous vetting). One also needs to evaluate the credibility of the medium (e.g., television, Internet, radio, social media, and book) and evaluate—not just accept without questioning—others' claims regarding the validity of a site, book, or other specific source of information. At this stage, one has to "make sense of information gathered from diverse sources by identifying misconceptions, main and supporting ideas, conflicting information, point of view, and biases" (American Association of School Librarians [AASL], 2009, p. 13) and conclude which sources/information are valid and accurate by using conscious strategies rather than simply using intuitive judgments or "rules of thumb." This phase is the most challenging segment of health information seeking and serves as a determinant of success (or lack thereof) in the information-seeking process. The following section on Sources of Health Information further explains this phase.

The fifth phase is *information management*, whereby one has to organize information that has been gathered in some manner to ensure easy retrieval and use in the future. The last phase is *information use*, in which one will synthesize information found across various resources, draw conclusions, and locate the answer to his or her original question and/ or the content that fulfills the information need. This phase also often involves implementation, such as using the information to solve a health problem; make health-related decisions; identify and engage in behaviors that will help a person to avoid health risks; share the health information found with family members and friends who may benefit from it; and advocate more broadly for personal, family, or community health.

THE IMPORTANCE OF HEALTH LITERACY

The conception of health has moved from a passive view (someone is either well or ill) to one that is more active and process based (someone is working toward preventing or managing disease). Hence, the dominant focus has shifted from doctors and treatments to patients and prevention, resulting in the need to strengthen our ability and confidence (as patients and consumers of health care) to look for, assess, understand, manage, share, adapt, and use health-related information. An individual's health literacy level has been found to predict his or her health status better than age, race, educational attainment, employment status, and income level (National Network of Libraries of Medicine, 2013). Greater health literacy also enables individuals to better communicate with health care providers such as doctors, nutritionists, and therapists, as they can pose more relevant, informed, and useful questions to health care providers. Another added advantage of greater health literacy is better information-seeking skills, not only for health but also in other domains, such as completing assignments for school.

SOURCES OF HEALTH INFORMATION: THE GOOD, THE BAD, AND THE IN-BETWEEN

For generations, doctors, nurses, nutritionists, health coaches, and other health professionals have been the trusted sources of health information. Additionally, researchers have found that young adults, when they have health-related questions, typically turn to a family member who has had firsthand experience with a health condition because of their family member's close proximity and because of their past experience with, and trust in, this individual. Expertise should be a core consideration when consulting a person, website, or book for health information. The credentials and background of the person or author and conflicting interests of the author (and his or her organization) must be checked and validated to ensure the likely credibility of the health information they are conveying. While books often have implied credibility because of the peer-review process involved, self-publishing has challenged this credibility, so qualifications of book authors should also be verified. When it comes to health information, currency of the source must also be examined. When examining health information/studies presented, pay attention to the exhaustiveness of research methods utilized to offer recommendations or conclusions. Small and nondiverse sample size is often—but not always—an indication of reduced credibility. Studies that confuse correlation with causation are another potential issue to watch for. Information seekers must also pay attention to the sponsors of the research studies. For example, if a study is sponsored by manufacturers of drug Y and the study recommends that drug Y is the best treatment to manage or cure a disease, this may indicate a lack of objectivity on the part of the researchers.

The Internet is rapidly becoming one of the main sources of health information. Online forums, news agencies, personal blogs, social media sites, pharmacy sites, and celebrity "doctors" are all offering medical and health information targeted to various types of people in regard to all types of diseases and symptoms. There are professional journalists, citizen journalists, hoaxers, and people paid to write fake health news on various sites that may appear to have a legitimate domain name and may even have authors who claim to have professional credentials, such as an MD. All these sites *may* offer useful information or information that appears to be useful and relevant; however, much of the information may be debatable and may fall into gray areas that require readers to discern credibility, reliability, and biases.

While broad recognition and acceptance of certain media, institutions, and people often serve as the most popular determining factors to assess credibility of health information among young people, keep in mind that there are legitimate Internet sites, databases, and books that publish health information and serve as sources of health information for doctors, other health sites, and members of the public. For example, MedlinePlus (https://medlineplus.gov) has trusted sources on over 975 diseases and conditions and presents the information in easy-to-understand language.

The chart here presents factors to consider when assessing credibility of health information. However, keep in mind that these factors function only as a guide and require continuous updating to keep abreast with the changes in the landscape of health information, information sources, and technologies.

The chart can serve as a guide; however, approaching a librarian about how one can go about assessing the credibility of both print and online

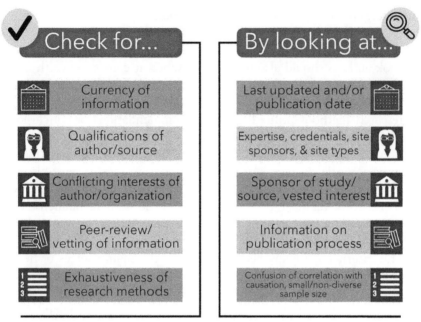

All images from flaticon.com

health information is far more effective than using generic checklist-type tools. While librarians are not health experts, they can apply and teach patrons strategies to determine the credibility of health information.

With the prevalence of fake sites and fake resources that appear to be legitimate, it is important to use the following health information assessment tips to verify health information that one has obtained (St. Jean et al., 2015, p. 151):

- **Don't assume you are right**: Even when you feel very sure about an answer, keep in mind that the answer may not be correct, and it is important to conduct (further) searches to validate the information.
- **Don't assume you are wrong**: You may actually have correct information, even if the information you encounter does not match—that is, you may be right and the resources that you have found may contain false information.
- **Take an open approach**: Maintain a critical stance by not including your preexisting beliefs as keywords (or letting them influence your choice of keywords) in a search, as this may influence what it is possible to find out.

- **Verify, verify, and verify**: Information found, especially on the Internet, needs to be validated, no matter how the information appears on the site (i.e., regardless of the appearance of the site or the quantity of information that is included).

Health literacy comes with experience navigating health information. Professional sources of health information, such as doctors, health care providers, and health databases, are still the best, but one also has the power to search for health information and then verify it by consulting with these trusted sources and by using the health information assessment tips and guide shared previously.

Mega Subramaniam, PhD
Associate Professor, College of Information
Studies, University of Maryland

REFERENCES AND FURTHER READING

American Association of School Librarians (AASL). (2009). *Standards for the 21st-century learner in action.* Chicago, IL: American Association of School Librarians.

Hilligoss, B., & Rieh, S.-Y. (2008). Developing a unifying framework of credibility assessment: Construct, heuristics, and interaction in context. *Information Processing & Management, 44*(4), 1467–1484.

Kuhlthau, C. C. (1988). Developing a model of the library search process: Cognitive and affective aspects. *Reference Quarterly, 28*(2), 232–242.

National Network of Libraries of Medicine (NNLM). (2013). Health literacy. Bethesda, MD: National Network of Libraries of Medicine. Retrieved from nnlm.gov/outreach/consumer/hlthlit.html

Ratzan, S. C., & Parker, R. M. (2000). Introduction. In C. R. Selden, M. Zorn, S. C. Ratzan, & R. M. Parker (Eds.), *National Library of Medicine current bibliographies in medicine: Health literacy.* NLM Pub. No. CBM 2000–1. Bethesda, MD: National Institutes of Health, U.S. Department of Health and Human Services.

St. Jean, B., Subramaniam, M., Taylor, N. G., Follman, R., Kodama, C., & Casciotti, D. (2015). The influence of positive hypothesis testing on youths' online health-related information seeking. *New Library World, 116*(3/4), 136–154.

St. Jean, B., Taylor, N. G., Kodama, C., & Subramaniam, M. (February 2017). Assessing the health information source perceptions of tweens using card-sorting exercises. *Journal of Information Science*, 44(2): 148–164. Retrieved from http://journals.sagepub.com/doi/abs/10.1177/0165551516687728

Subramaniam, M., St. Jean, B., Taylor, N. G., Kodama, C., Follman, R., & Casciotti, D. (2015). Bit by bit: Using design-based research to improve the health literacy of adolescents. *JMIR Research Protocols*, 4(2), paper e62. Retrieved from http://www.ncbi.nlm.nih.gov/pmc/articles/PMC4464334/

Valenza, J. (2016, November 26). Truth, truthiness, and triangulation: A news literacy toolkit for a "post-truth" world [Web log]. Retrieved from http://blogs.slj.com/neverendingsearch/2016/11/26/truth-truthiness-triangulation-and-the-librarian-way-a-news-literacy-toolkit-for-a-post-truth-world/

Common Misconceptions about Food Labels

1. THE SERVING SIZE GIVEN ON A FOOD LABEL IS A RECOMMENDATION ON HOW MUCH OF THAT FOOD PEOPLE SHOULD CONSUME

Perhaps because "serving size" is given on the Nutrition Facts panel along with dietary recommendations, consumers assume that the serving size itself is some sort of recommendation as well. However, on the food label, serving size simply provides a unit of measure so that consumers can apply the other information on the Nutrition Facts panel. In other words, if the Nutrition Facts panel states that a product such as fruit jelly contains 7 grams of added sugar, the consumer needs to know how much of the jelly contains 7 grams of added sugar. The FDA (U.S. Food and Drug Administration) determines what serving size should be used for each category of food product, and aims to make serving sizes similar to what people generally consume. To learn more about serving size regulations and what serving size means on food labels, see Question 10.

2. THE % DAILY VALUE FIGURES ON THE NUTRITION FACTS PANEL ARE PRECISE VALUES THAT APPLY TO EVERYONE

Values for many food components listed on the Nutrition Facts panel are provided in both measures of weight (e.g., grams or milligrams) and % Daily Value. Both can be very helpful, but unless people know their daily target for a given nutrient or other food component, the % Daily Value is more useful than the measure of weight. The % Daily Value figures are derived from a table of nutrition recommendations designed by the FDA. The Daily Values table in turn is based on more complete nutrition tables that list nutrition requirements for 22 different population groups based on age, sex, and for women, the conditions of pregnancy and lactation. The Daily Values used on most food labels are for everyone four years of age and older, but they were drawn from the values for adult men and women, 19–30 years old. While nutrition requirements for some nutrients vary little across the 22 categories, others, such as recommendations for iron intake, vary quite a bit. To learn more about the Daily Values, see Question 9.

3. FOOD LABEL REGULATIONS ARE REVIEWED AND UPDATED ON A REGULAR SCHEDULE

The regulations governing what information must appear, and what information may not appear, on food labels undergo continual revision. These regulations rest in great part with two federal agencies: the U.S. Food and Drug Administration (FDA) and the U.S. Department of Agriculture (USDA). Unlike public health documents, such as Healthy People or the U.S. Dietary Guidelines, that are revised every five years when an ad hoc committee of experts is invited to review and rewrite them, the FDA and USDA are working every day to carry out their many functions, including the regulation of food labels. Food label regulations are not reviewed and updated on a regular schedule, and rarely in any systematic fashion. Instead, changes in food label regulations are set in motion by a variety of unpredictable factors. For more information on how the food label is updated, see Question 6.

4. ALL CLAIMS APPEARING ON FOOD LABELS ARE REGULATED AND HAVE A CLEAR MEANING

Many parts of a food product's label are regulated, in the United States primarily by the FDA. The FDA has developed extensive regulations regarding what information must be included on food labels, and what statements may and may not appear on food packages, with the goal that food labels should be truthful and not misleading. Thus, it is natural for people to assume that all parts of a food label conform to some group of regulations. However, only some of the information appearing on food labels is regulated and has a clear meaning. A food's packaging displays a combination of marketing and regulated label components. To learn more about how the information on food labels is regulated, see Question 1.

5. EVERY LABELED FOOD PRODUCT IS TESTED IN A LABORATORY TO DETERMINE ITS CALORIC AND NUTRIENT VALUES AS LISTED ON THE NUTRITION FACTS PANEL

Most people assume the Nutrition Facts panel, listing the product's calories and nutrition information, must display the actual calorie and nutrient values from that particular product, and assume that the product itself was tested in some kind of laboratory to determine its exact calorie content and nutrient values. In fact, many food products have never seen the inside of a food laboratory. Only the largest food product producers have laboratories routinely used for product analysis. Smaller companies can pay an outside laboratory to analyze their products, but most opt for using standard nutrient values for the product's food ingredients, using the food product's recipe.

Readers can learn more about the accuracy of the caloric and nutrient values listed on a product's Nutrition Facts panel by reading the answer to Question 5.

QUESTIONS AND ANSWERS

Regulation of Food Labels

I. How are food labels regulated in the United States?

Food labels are primarily regulated in the United States by two federal agencies: the U.S. Food and Drug Administration (FDA) and the U.S. Department of Agriculture (USDA). A little familiarity with these organizations can help consumers get a better understanding of how to interpret food labels.

The FDA regulates labeling of over 80% of food products and oversees food labels for all processed foods created and sold in the United States. It regulates labeling for meat from "exotic" animals, such as alligator and venison; all seafood; and bioengineered food.

As the name implies, the FDA oversees not only food but also drugs. Specifically, it is responsible for regulating the following products:

- Food (excludes meat and poultry, which are regulated by the USDA)
- Beverages (excludes alcohol)
- Tobacco
- Cosmetics (although they do not require FDA approval before entering the market, the FDA researches products and acts when they are found to be harmful)
- Human and veterinary drugs (both prescription and nonprescription)
- Medical devices (from tongue depressors to pacemakers)

- Biological products, such as vaccines, blood, and tissue
- Products that emit radiation, such as ultraviolet lights for tanning and medical imaging devices

The FDA interacts with a number of other agencies in overseeing food labels. For example:

- Pesticides: The Environmental Protection Agency (EPA) regulates pesticides, but the FDA regularly tests for elevated levels of pesticides in food.
- Water: The FDA regulates bottled water, while the EPA sets standards for local drinking water.
- Dietary supplements: Until 1994, dietary supplements were regulated similarly to foods. However, the Dietary Supplement Health and Education Act gave the manufacturer the responsibility for assuring the safety, efficacy, and truthful labeling of dietary supplements. Once the product is available to consumers, the FDA is responsible for proving a dietary supplement unsafe if it has concerns. The FDA regulates labeling of dietary supplements.

The FDA works with the Centers for Disease Control and Prevention (CDC) when an outbreak of foodborne illness occurs. The CDC is a federal agency that "conducts and supports health promotion, prevention and preparedness activities" in the United States in order to improve public health. The FDA does not inspect restaurants, but its Food Code is used by city and state health departments who do the inspections. The Food Code is designed to guide establishments on keeping food safe to eat and to prevent foodborne infections.

The FDA works with the Federal Trade Commission (FTC) when the advertising on food packages (as well as other advertising for food and other products) is misleading and/or fraudulent. The mission of the FTC is to protect consumers by stopping "unfair, deceptive, or fraudulent practices in the marketplace." It investigates companies when consumers or agencies like the FDA file complaints.

The FDA is divided into many departments to fulfill all of these functions. The Center for Food Safety and Applied Nutrition (CFSAN) is the branch of the FDA that regulates food labeling. Its mission is to make sure the foods people eat in the United States "are safe, wholesome, sanitary, and properly labeled." The FDA strives to ensure that labels are truthful and not misleading.

In terms of food labels, the USDA mainly oversees labeling of meat and poultry, as well as egg products. (However, the FDA regulates food labels for whole eggs in their shells.) The USDA also oversees the USDA Organic food label and use of the term "natural," and many terms related to animal treatment used on labels. Like the FDA, the USDA has many branches and performs a variety of functions. Its primary goals are to support the U.S. agricultural economy and "provide a safe, sufficient, and nutritious food supply for the American people." Some of the most important areas of the USDA include the following:

- Food safety and labeling: The USDA administers food safety and inspection programs for the foods it oversees, as well as labeling and packaging regulations.
- Organic program: All farms, wild crop harvesting and handling operations that wish to display the USDA organic label on their agricultural products, must meet the USDA's National Organic Program standards.
- Food and nutrition aid services: The USDA provides nutrition aid programs, including the Special Supplemental Nutrition Program for Women, Infants, and Children and the Supplemental Nutrition Assistance Program (food stamps) program. These programs provide economic assistance for purchasing food for low-income households.
- Food and nutrition policy and education: The USDA generates the production of several important policy documents. For example, the Dietary Guidelines for Americans (DGA) document, updated every five years, comes from the USDA. The DGA helps guide FDA and USDA food labeling, as well as many other important initiatives. The USDA's website ChooseMyPlate.gov (referred to as "MyPlate") diet planning guidelines and information also comes from the USDA.
- Marketing and regulatory programs: The USDA helps set national and international standards for agricultural marketing. It also oversees animal and plant health inspection and regulates meatpacking and stockyards.
- Farm and foreign agricultural services: Several USDA departments administer programs that strive to support U.S. farmers and ranchers. Programs provide assistance for enhancing domestic production of agricultural products; marketing U.S. agricultural products to other countries; and credit, disaster, and emergency assistance.

- Rural development: Support for rural development includes economic support for water and sewage systems, housing, health clinics, and utilities in rural areas.
- Research, education, and economics: The USDA generates research and reports that help guide policy, strategy, and regulation.

In addition to the oversight provided by the FDA and USDA, a number of third-party verification logos may be used on food labels. (Third party means that the organization certifying the food product is not the manufacturer or the government.) To display these third-party verification endorsements, the food producer generally submits its product and pays a fee to the third-party organization. A site visit may also be required. If the product meets the standards of the certifying organization, the product may then display the logo on the food label. For example, stamps or logos certifying foods as kosher or non-genetically modified organisms are provided by third-party organizations.

States may also regulate food labeling. For example, sell-by and use-by labeling is regulated by states. Milk and milk products are often regulated by state dairy boards. States must comply with federal regulations regarding food labeling.

2. What is the history of food label regulations in the United States?

The evolution of food labeling in the United States occurred alongside efforts of scientists, food producers, and consumers to improve the safety and quality of food and drugs. In the mid-1800s, many people became concerned with food safety and the adulteration of food and drugs being sold in the United States. At this time, a lack of regulation led to frequent adulteration, contamination, and false advertising of a wide variety of goods. Medications containing opium and cocaine were sold over the counter without warning labels or ingredient lists, and completely innocuous substances were marketed as the cure for various diseases and symptoms. Foods were often contaminated with toxic chemicals and colors, or were not the products they were stated to be. For example, products claiming to be "fruit" jams were made with water, glucose, grass seed, and artificial color.

Food producers wanted standardization of weights and measures, and inspections to establish product quality to improve product sales. Many states had their own regulations, which made trade difficult for producers wanting to sell their products in more than one state.

In response to these concerns, Congress passed the Pure Food and Drugs Act in 1906, which prohibited interstate commerce in contaminated and misbranded food and drugs. Federal regulation was overseen by the Chemistry Division of the U.S. Department of Agriculture (USDA), which in 1930 became the Food and Drug Administration (FDA). The authority of the FDA was later expanded through the 1938 Federal Food, Drug, and Cosmetic Act to cover a wider range of products and manufacturing standards.

Efforts to regulate and standardize food labels grew throughout the 20th century. Product names continued to become legally defined. For example, the Oleomargarine Act, passed in 1950, mandated the labeling of colored oleomargarine to distinguish it from butter. Today consumers know that "fruit drinks" are different from "fruit juice." Ingredient lists became required and regulated. For example, in 1958, the Food Additives Amendment was passed, requiring manufacturers to establish the safety of new food additives, and list all additives on food labels. Net quantity had to be declared on package labels. Food labels had to include information on manufacturers and distributors. Imported foods were required to list the country of origin.

During the 1970s scientific research on the associations between nutrition and chronic disease, especially heart disease, became a focus of national public health campaigns. In 1980 the USDA published its first version of its Dietary Guidelines for Americans, and consumers were encouraged to give more consideration to their food choices. Standardized and mandatory nutrition information debuted on food labels in 1994, following the passage of the Nutrition Labeling and Education Act (NLEA) in 1990. The NLEA required nutrition labeling on all packaged food, and all health claims on packages be standardized. Today's food label is very similar to the 1994 food label design.

During the following two decades, several changes to food labels were mandated. One of the most striking came in 2003, when the FDA announced that labels must include trans-fat content as part of the Nutrition Facts panel. Researchers had established evidence that trans-fat intake was associated with a greater risk of cardiovascular disease.

The USDA regulates labeling of meat and poultry. In 2012, the USDA updated meat labels to include nutrition information. These labels are required on packages for all ground or chopped meat products, such as ground beef, ground turkey, and ground pork. Labels are also mandated for 40 of the most popular cuts of single-ingredient, raw meat and poultry products. These labels may appear either on the package itself or as a display at point of purchase.

After a long period of research and discussion, the FDA announced new rules for the Nutrition Facts panel in May 2016. The changes reflected continuing concern about rising obesity rates and associated chronic health problems that accompany obesity and a poor diet, including type 2 diabetes, hypertension, and cardiovascular disease. Changes to the Nutrition Facts panel included the following:

- More prominent information on calorie content: The larger type size for the word "Calories" and the number of calories, as well as bolding the font for number of calories and serving size were designed to encourage consumers to become more aware of their calorie intake.
- More realistic serving sizes: Serving sizes for several food and beverage categories have changed to reflect actual consumption practices. For example, a serving of soda increased from 8 oz to 12 oz, since 12 oz is the size of a typical container (and actual serving). Some packages must include calories per container as well as calories per serving.
- Information on added sugars: Instead of featuring only the amount of total sugars, the new label also spells out how much sugar is added to the product. More recent dietary guidelines have encouraged consumers to consume less sugar, especially less added sugars.
- Clearer information on nutrient content: The new label reflects updated Daily Values (DV) and, in addition to %DV for listed nutrients, lists the actual amount of each nutrient in a serving.
- Change in featured nutrients: The Nutrition Facts panel includes information on several key nutrients commonly low in diets—vitamin D, calcium, iron, and potassium. Low levels of these nutrients have been associated with numerous health problems. Vitamins A and C were featured on the old label, but have been removed, since deficiencies in these nutrients are less common.

3. What foods are not required to have nutrition facts labels, and why?

The Nutrition Labeling and Education Act of 1990 and subsequent revisions spell out which foods must bear which types of labels and which foods are exempt from nutrition label regulations (see Question 2). Some foods are not required to bear nutrition facts labels. These foods include all types of seafood, as well as raw vegetables and fruits. Ready-to-eat foods are also not required to bear nutrition facts labels. Examples of ready-to-eat foods include products from delicatessens and bakeries.

Vendors selling foods on the sidewalk or in settings such as festivals are not required to have labels on their foods.

The reason no nutrition labels are required on these foods is that the Food and Drug Administration (FDA) has determined that requiring labels would be excessively difficult for the people and companies selling these products. Such products and their production are still required by the FDA and other local, state, and federal agencies to be clean, safe, and prepared following certain guidelines governing food sanitation and worker safety.

Meat and poultry, whose safety and labeling is governed by the U.S. Department of Agriculture (USDA), has its own set of labeling requirements, as described in Question 1. The USDA requires the Nutrition Facts panel on all individual packages of ground and chopped meat products, such as ground beef, ground turkey, and ground lamb. Labeling is also mandated for 40 of the most popular cuts of single-ingredient, raw meat, and poultry products, such as beef loin sirloin steak, pork loin chops, and chicken breasts. However, the Nutrition Facts panel may appear either on individual packages for these or as a display at point of purchase.

Small business meat producers and sellers are exempt from these regulations, however. Small businesses are those who employ 500 or fewer people, and sell less than 100,000 lbs of the product in question per year. So, for example, an independently owned local store with a meat department is probably exempt. However, if a product's label makes a nutrition statement or claim, the Nutrition Facts panel is required, to help consumers understand the label information. Similarly, stores that slice and weigh meat for consumers are exempt from labeling those products. Small facilities that slaughter, process, and package meat generally do not need labels on their products, nor do producers that sell whole-animal carcasses. The USDA has determined that applying the labeling rules in these cases would be an unfair burden.

Some categories of food products must have packaging labels but are exempt from nutrition facts labeling. These food packages must still display all required information (statement of identity; net quantity of contents; ingredient list; and the name and address of the manufacturer, packer, or distributor), but it need not include nutrition information. Foods that contain insignificant amounts (close to or equal to zero) of all nutrients that require listing do not need labels. An example of a food meeting this exemption is coffee. A package of coffee will still list all other required information, but is not required to list nutrient facts. A similar example is packaging for food dyes.

Foods with total packaging surface area that is less than 12 square inches are not required to display nutrition facts. For example, a small bottle of a condiment such as hot sauce is not required to include nutrition facts.

Small businesses manufacturing food products may also be exempt from nutrition food labeling requirements. The FDA defines a small business based on its annual sales volume. Low volume of sales of food products from larger businesses may also be exempt, but the company selling the product may have to request an exemption from the FDA if it is of a certain size.

However, even products from small businesses and low-volume food products are required to include labels under certain conditions. If the food makes a nutrient claim either in the food packaging or in the product's advertising, it must have a Nutrition Facts panel. For example, if the manufacturer advertises the food as "low fat," "low sodium," or "gluten free," it must have the standard Nutrition Facts panel.

Interestingly, many products that are technically exempt from nutrition labeling still voluntarily include this information on their labels. Some do this because their sales are growing and the company is anticipating reaching a sales volume that will require labels. (Once a product's sales reach a certain level, the company has 18 months to meet FDA nutrition labeling requirements.) Other manufacturers include the information to satisfy consumers.

Small manufacturers that sell their product in large stores are required to have Nutrition Fact panels on their products. So small manufacturers that wish to sell their products through major grocery store chains must include Nutrition Fact panels on their product labels.

What can consumers do if they need nutrition information on products with no nutrition facts labels? For example, people trying to limit sodium who consume a bagel every morning from a bakery on their way to work might wish to know the sodium content of their bagel.

Consumers whose diet regularly includes unlabeled foods and who need nutrition information have a few options. Large producers and sellers may list nutrition information on a website accessible to consumers. For example, the Bruegger's Bagels website (https://www.nutrition-charts .com/brueggers-bagels-nutrition-information/) says that most of its bagels contain about 500 mg of sodium.

If this information is not available, consumers can find the nutrition information for standard or comparable products on the USDA website (https://ndb.nal.usda.gov/ndb/). For example, according to the USDA website, a standard bagel (81 g) contains 291 mg of sodium. Many bagels, including the Bruegger's Bagels described earlier, are larger than this, so consumers must pay attention to serving size when interpreting this information, as product sizes can vary considerably.

4. What information is required on food labels?

Both the U.S. Food and Drug Administration (FDA) and the U.S. Department of Agriculture (USDA) require a specific set of basic information on the food labels they oversee (see Question 1). Both agencies require the following on labels of packaged food available for sale to consumers:

1. Name of the product. Many names are regulated, so that the product's name accurately reflects the food's content and production process. For example, some products that may look similar to cheese must be called "cheese food" or "cheese product" to differentiate it from true cheese.
2. Net quantity of the product. This means the amount of the product, by weight, in the package, not including the weight of the package. USDA labels (most meat and poultry) require the weight in English measures such as pounds or ounces. FDA labels (most other foods) must provide the weight in both English and metric (kilograms or grams) units.
3. Ingredient list. All ingredients must be listed in order, from the greatest to the lowest in weight. There are a few exceptions, however. For example, some food colorings and flavorings do not need to be listed, except as "artificial coloring" or "artificial flavoring." Others must be listed by name, such as FD&C Yellow No. 5, since this coloring can cause hives in a small minority of consumers. Individual spices need not be listed, and the label may simply include "spices." Interestingly, caffeine only needs to appear on the ingredient list if caffeine itself is added to the food. If caffeine is a natural component of another ingredient, for example, coffee (as in coffee ice cream), caffeine need not be listed as an ingredient.
4. Name of the manufacturer or distributor, along with the town, state, and zip code of the location. If the business is easy to find, for example, if it is listed in an accessible directory of some sort, the full street address is not required. However, the street address is required if information on the exact location would be hard to find, or if the business has multiple locations and it might be difficult to determine which is the primary address. A mailing address such as a post office box in lieu

of a street address is not permitted. The exact location must be listed in case someone needs to find the business.

5. Country of origin. Imported products must list the country of origin. On packaged food regulated by the FDA, labels may bear a statement such as "Product of Denmark." The USDA also requires country of origin on many products, including fresh and frozen fruits and vegetables, as well as some types of nuts. For products with no packaging, country or origin may appear on a sticker on the food; this is the case for bananas, which might bear a sticker saying "Costa Rica." Avocadoes might show a sticker with "Product of Mexico." Some fresh fruits and vegetables that are sold loose may show country of origin on a sign at the point of purchase.

6. Serving size and number of servings contained in the package. These appear on products with the Nutrition Facts panel on both FDA- and USDA-regulated packaged foods.

7. Nutrition facts, primarily the Nutrition Facts panel. The Nutrition Facts panel is required on almost all FDA-regulated food package labels. The USDA requires the Nutrition Facts panel on most packaged meat and poultry labels found in large stores. (For more information on which foods do not require labels, see Question 3.) The Nutrition Facts panel displays a great deal of nutrition information in a compact format. Question 7 and the following section discuss the Nutrition Facts panel in greater detail.

8. Food allergens. Foods containing one or more of eight common allergens must list these prominently on the label.

Many other requirements govern food labels, depending on food product ingredients, food processing and manufacturing methods, and label claims. For example, if a food contains the fat replacer olestra, the package is required to state this on the label. Foods containing raw or not ready-to-eat meat or poultry must include this fact on the label. If foods are packaged under pressure, their label must indicate that contents are under pressure. Whole foods that have been irradiated must include the radura symbol on the label, and the phrase "treated with radiation" or "treated by irradiation." Yet, if irradiated ingredients are part of a food product that has not been irradiated, no label is required.

Much of the language used on labels is regulated but not required. For example, the USDA regulates words such as "certified," "free range or free roaming," "fresh," "frozen," "halal," "kosher," and "natural." Grades of meat are also regulated by the USDA. The FDA regulates wording that implies a nutrient claim. The terms "fat free," "low fat," "less fat," and "light," for example, all have strict and clear definitions. Similarly, the FDA also closely regulates health claims. For example, the statement "Adequate calcium and vitamin D as part of a healthful diet, along with physical activity, may reduce the risk of osteoporosis in later life" is an FDA-approved health claim.

5. How accurate is the information on food labels?

The most important thing to remember about food product packages is that some components must conform to label regulations, but much of it does not. Logos and banners that look like official statements often appear on packaging. But in truth, they are simply advertising: pictures of foods, farms, and other images do their best to lure hungry or hurried shoppers. For example, mouth-watering pictures of fruit may be featured on labels of beverages that contain no fruit whatsoever. Banners with claims such as "fresh fruit flavor!" are unregulated and may appear on products that do not contain real fruit. This advertising can be extremely misleading.

Educated consumers understand which components of food labels are most apt to deliver trustworthy information. These are the components described in the previous question (Question 4). While a picture of fruit may dominate the food packaging, consumers can check the ingredient list to see whether fruit actually makes it into the food product's recipe.

One of the most important food label accuracy issues concerns food allergens, since food allergies can cause life-threatening emergencies. The Food and Drug Administration (FDA) does inspect a variety of foods as part of its regulatory work. In addition, consumers themselves may bring complaints about food products suspected of causing allergic reactions to the attention of the FDA. Over 100 food products are recalled each year due to the undeclared presence of the eight most common food allergens. This fact is quite alarming to people with severe food allergies, who may be reluctant to use very many food products, relying instead on the foods they know to be safe. A company with mislabeled products may be subject to criminal penalties, civil sanctions, or both.

The nutrition information required by the FDA and U.S. Department of Agriculture (USDA) on food labels provides rough estimates that are helpful to most people. However, consumers should know that the information on the Nutrition Facts panel is permitted to be within a 20% margin of error. In other words, a food stating that it contains 300 calories per serving might be as low as 240 or as high as 360 calories. Similarly, values for any given nutrient are allowed a similar variability. A stated calcium content of 200 mg could be anywhere from 160 mg to 240 mg. A protein content of 10 g might be somewhere between 8 g and 12 g.

Why is the range so large?

The nutrition content of any given type of food varies considerably because of a number of factors, including the soil and growing conditions, ripeness at the time of harvest, an animal's diet, length and conditions of storage, food processing methods, and more. As an example, since the potassium content of individual oranges varies the potassium content of orange juice will vary as well. The 20% margin of error allows food manufacturers to give consumers average figures without testing each batch of a food product: an impossible and very costly undertaking. Studies suggest that the calorie values on food labels, on average, tend to be just a little under actual values, about 4% to 8% low.

Do labels need approval before a labeled product is put on the market?

Food producers and manufacturers bear the responsibility for honest and accurate food labels. The FDA is not required to approve any food labels before a product goes to market. Only a very few labels need approval from the USDA before the product is put on the market; most food producers are able to use a generically approved label that does not need further evaluation. Companies are supposed to follow the legal guidelines laid out by the FDA and USDA.

It is in a food producer's best interest to comply with the law. While the FDA does not perform systematic policing of labels, it does catch some errors, and dishonest or misleading labels can be brought to its attention, or to the attention of the Federal Trade Commission, by consumer groups. In such cases, products may be seized or removed from the market, and law suits can ensue, costing companies large amounts of money and damaging their reputations and the reputations of their products.

6. What is the process for updating the food label?

The Food and Drug Administration (FDA) and, to a lesser extent, the U.S. Department of Agriculture (USDA) are continually revising food label regulations. They create new rules and update existing ones as the perceived need arises. They are prompted to do so by their own research, as well as petitions from food companies, consumer groups, scientific advisory groups, and a wide variety of other organizations.

Records of the adoption or revision of regulations regarding food labels may be found in the *Federal Register* (federalregister.gov). The *Federal Register* is the daily record of the federal government. It is published each business day by the National Archives and Records Administration's Office of the Federal Register. The *Federal Register* records federal agency actions, including creation of regulations; proposed rules and notices of interest to the public; and executive orders, proclamations, and other documents. In general, when considering an update to food label regulations, the FDA publishes a notice regarding its intentions, sends out a call for comments, considers the feedback it receives, then publishes a ruling. This whole process can take years, depending on the complexity of the proposed regulation.

An interesting example is a revision made by the FDA to regulations regarding the use of the word "healthy" on food labels in 2016. The original rules for defining the word "healthy" included the requirement that the food have no more than 3 g of total fat per serving, with only 1 g of that as saturated fat. These rules reflected older nutrition recommendations. Over time, newer nutrition guidelines, such as the USDA's Dietary Guidelines for Americans, evolved to focus less on total fat and more on types of fat. Instead of urging people to limit all fats, the Dietary Guidelines shifted to urging people to limit saturated and trans fats. Ironically, according to the old "healthy" guidelines, products such as sugary pastries and breakfast cereals could be labeled "healthy," while foods like nuts and avocadoes could not.

The following summary quotation from the *Federal Register* provides a good illustration of the process for updating the food label: The FDA "is amending the regulation authorizing a health claim on the relationship between dietary saturated fat and cholesterol and risk of coronary heart disease (CHD) to permit raw fruits and vegetables that fail to comply with the 'low fat' definition and/or the minimum nutrient content requirement to be eligible to bear the claim. We are taking this action in response to a petition submitted by the American Heart Association (the petitioner). The amendment expands the use of this health claim to certain fruits and vegetables that are currently ineligible for the health claim." The FDA welcomed and read comments, and then updated the food label rule accordingly.

The part of the food label that is the most complicated and helpful, but is rarely updated, is the Nutrition Facts panel. The Nutrition Facts panel began as an optional component of the food label in 1973. At this time, the FDA mandated a Nutrition Facts panel only on a food label when the label or advertising of that product made a nutrition claim, or if nutrients were added to the food. The label needed to list the following required nutrients, and the amount of each expressed in units per usual serving: number of calories, protein, carbohydrate, fat, vitamin A, vitamin C, thiamin, riboflavin, niacin, calcium, and iron. Values for sodium, saturated fatty acids, and polyunsaturated fatty acids were optional.

Many labels with this early Nutrition Facts panel presented nutrients as percentages of the U.S. Recommended Daily Allowances (U.S. RDAs). The FDA used 1968 values from standard National Academies of Sciences RDA tables to create a precursor table to the Daily Values that are used on food labels today. The FDA used the highest value for each nutrient in the RDA tables for adult males and adult nonpregnant, nonlactating females. The 1968 Daily Values remained the standard used on food labels until the recent changes mandated in 2016.

With the passage of the Nutrition Labeling and Education Act in 1990, Congress gave the FDA stronger authority and required nutrition labeling on most food packages. The FDA spent two years designing the final regulations, hearing comments from scientists, consumers, food producers, and many other groups. The FDA was careful to design food label requirements in ways that would encourage consumers to follow other government nutrition recommendations, such as the Dietary Guidelines for Americans published by the USDA. A new group of required nutrients was set for the new Nutrition Facts panel. This panel is very similar to the Nutrition Facts panel on food labels today. Except for the addition of trans fat to the list in 1999, the label remained unchanged until then-president of the United States Barack Obama called for an update to the Nutrition Facts panel in 2016 as part of a package of measures to help address increasing rates of obesity in the United States.

As before, the procedures for the updating of the food label rested with the FDA. The FDA listened to concerns from all constituents: other governmental agencies, scientific groups, consumer groups, and food manufacturers. The FDA changed several features on the Nutrition Facts panel to try to present the most important information consumers needed to know to make purchasing and food choice decisions.

It is not hard to imagine that the FDA rules never please everyone, and must often be a compromise. For example, food producers do not want to highlight information that might influence consumers to not choose their products. Consumers might want testing of products in ways that are prohibitively expensive to producers, and reduce competition in the marketplace. Scientists have charged that the USDA's Dietary Guidelines for

Americans, which help guide FDA food label policies, are unduly influenced by USDA's constituencies (farmers, ranchers, and other food producers). Large corporations influenced by a given regulation may exert strong pressure on the FDA to push their interests forward. For most people, the food label regulations will never be perfect, but hopefully they can help a majority of citizens much of the time.

Nutrition Facts Panel

7. Who regulates the Nutrition Facts panel, and why is it so important?

The Nutrition Facts panel is regulated by the U.S. Food and Drug Administration (FDA). It is one of the most important parts of the label because it provides consumers with the best information regarding the nutritional composition of the labeled food product.

The Nutrition Facts panel was created in response to increasing concern about the meaning of label claims along with increasing consumer interest in nutrition. Public interest in the association between nutrition and health blossomed in the late 1980s, as scientific research began to suggest strong links between diet and health. Early research found an association between certain dietary components and heart disease. Over the years, research focus expanded to include associations between diet and many other health concerns, including high blood pressure, type 2 diabetes, osteoporosis, obesity, intestinal health, and certain types of cancer. More recently, diet has been suggested to influence immune system function, as well as risk of developing dementia, depression, and anxiety.

Food manufacturers have taken advantage of this consumer interest and have shaped products and their labels to appeal to the consumer drive to purchase healthful products. The U.S. Congress and the FDA responded to the increasing number of health claims on food products by increasing their regulation. While the Nutrition Facts panel began as an optional component of the food label in 1973, with the passage of the

Nutrition Labeling and Education Act in 1990, the U.S. Congress mandated that a Nutrition Facts panel be included on almost all packaged food products. Congress, and many groups throughout the country, hoped that the Nutrition Facts panel would improve transparency between label health and nutrition claims and actual nutritional composition of foods.

The Nutrition Facts panel is helpful to consumers for several reasons. First, as the FDA originally intended, it can help consumers find the nutrition information implied by label claims. While many label health and nutrition claims are regulated by the FDA, very few consumers know what these claims, such as "low-fat" or "light," actually mean in terms of food composition. And many statements appearing on labels are unregulated. With the information provided by the Nutrition Facts panel, consumers reading a claim such as "low sodium" are able to easily find out how much sodium is actually contained in a serving of the product. Consumers can also quickly see how much of their daily sodium limit is contained in that serving. When shoppers see "excellent source of protein," they can check the Nutrition Facts panel to find out how much protein is really in a serving.

Second, the Nutrition Facts panel provides people with information they need because of dietary restrictions or health concerns. Many people are on special diets, or seeking certain nutrient intakes. For example, some people are counseled to include a certain amount of calcium and vitamin D in their diets to prevent or treat low bone density issues. These consumers may be keeping track of how many milligrams of calcium and how many micrograms of vitamin D they consume each daily. The Nutrition Facts panel provides this information.

Third, the transparency provided by the Nutrition Facts panel encourages food manufacturers to reformulate (and hopefully improve the quality of) their products. This occurred when trans fat amounts became required on food labels. Companies quickly transitioned to other ingredients and manufacturing methods to lower the amount of trans fat in their products, since these amounts would now appear on their labels and possibly discourage consumers from purchasing these products. Food manufacturers responded in a similar fashion when added sugars became required on the Nutrition Facts panel, changing the sugar content of their recipes.

8. How do food manufacturers figure out the nutrient values for the Nutrition Facts panel on their product labels?

A food manufacturer has two basic options for figuring out the nutrient values of a given food product and designing a label that is compliant with Food and Drug Administration (FDA) labeling regulations. The first option is sending a sample of the food product to a laboratory that performs nutrient testing. These laboratories are equipped with the complex instrumentation needed to perform chemical analyses for all of the nutrients required on the Nutrition Facts panel and can determine a food product's nutrient values. The second method is to calculate a food's nutrient values from the nutrient values of the ingredients. These values can be found in a number of databases. Food manufacturers use these two methods in a variety of ways.

Some very large manufacturers have their own food analysis laboratories in-house. An in-house food laboratory is very expensive to create and maintain, but can make financial sense for a very large company that requires a lot of testing for new products and labels. Large companies are continually creating new food products, and the ones going to market will need accurate labels. Easy access to nutrition analysis is also helpful for companies trying to formulate products to achieve a certain nutrient composition. They can check and see if their recipe is adequate to meet standards for a given nutrient content claim. For example, they may wish to know whether the sodium content of the product meets the standards for a "low in sodium" nutrient content claim. Or a new formulation may be required to meet FDA regulations. For example, a manufacturer may need to reduce the amount of trans fat in a product and want to test a variety of recipes to achieve this for a given product.

A number of commercial food laboratories are not part of any single company but sell their services to any food manufacturer. In addition to testing a product for nutrient values, these businesses often offer other helpful options to food manufacturers, such as advice on recipes, label formatting, allergen statements, and advice on which nutrient or health claims could appear on the label. A company preparing to market a new food can send a sample to the food laboratory and receive the results. This process can take a few weeks and can cost several hundred dollars per product. Therefore, a manufacturer planning to market several products, perhaps several variations of a similar product, may pay several thousand dollars to have all of their products tested in a food laboratory.

Most companies opt for calculating nutrient values of their products by adding up the nutrient values of the product ingredients. A variety of databases are available for these calculations. For example, the U.S. Department of Agriculture database of nutrient values includes information on over 7,600 foods and is partially updated each year. Their values are obtained from their own laboratories as well as commercial laboratories and food producers themselves. Many commercial databases are even larger.

A food product manufacturer can elect to use ingredient nutrient information in one of three ways. The manufacturer may simply hire a consultant from an independent company to perform the nutrient content calculations and advise on other labeling details. Some manufacturers buy their own nutrition analysis software packages that give them access to useful databases and label designs. And many manufacturers buy licenses to web-based nutrition analysis software. This is the cheapest option and is rapidly becoming the most popular. The software uses the food recipe to calculate nutrient values, produce the Nutrition Facts panel for the product, write allergen statements, and identify nutrient content claims the manufacturer is eligible to include.

9. What are Daily Values, and what does % Daily Value mean?

The Daily Values are a set of dietary standards used on food labels to help consumers understand the nutrient content of food products. The percent (%) Daily Value tells consumers what percentage of a Daily Value is supplied by one serving of the labeled food product. For example, if a food product label shows that the product serving contains "Fiber 3g 10%," consumers would know that if they eat one serving of that product, they would meet 10% of their recommended daily fiber requirements. The % Daily Value figures are helpful because they help consumers understand how much they should eat of certain nutrients. The figures also help consumers compare similar food products and make informed choices. In general, foods supplying 20% or more of a given nutrient per serving are considered to be "high" in that nutrient; foods that supply 5% or less of the Daily Value for a given nutrient in one serving are considered to be "low" in that nutrient.

The Daily Values are created by the Food and Drug Administration (FDA) and are drawn from established nutrition tables. Nutrition agencies from the United States and Canada have compiled recommended intake level for a variety of nutrients for 22 different population groups, based on age and sex, and, for women, conditions of pregnancy and lactation. The complete set of these tables is extremely large and obviously does not fit on the label of a food product.

To create the Daily Values for most vitamins and minerals, the FDA used the highest value for each nutrient in the nutrition tables for adult males and adult nonpregnant, nonlactating females. In the United States these nutrient reference values are set by the Food and Nutrition Board of the Health and Medicine Division of the National Academies of Sciences, Engineering, and Medicine (NASEM). NASEM is a nonprofit, nongovernmental organization whose goal is to provide unbiased, authoritative advice on issues relating to health and medicine. Scientists serving on NASEM are volunteers, nominated by their peers because of their scientific achievements and recognition.

There are actually four sets of Daily Values. The values appearing on labels for most packaged foods are for adults and children four years of age and older. But there are also Daily Values for (1) infants 1–12 months, (2) children 1–3 years old, and (3) pregnant and lactating women. These values are only used on food products specifically designed for these groups.

The Daily Values for adults and children over age four are based on a 2,000-calorie daily intake. Calorie intakes that are much higher or lower would change recommendations for grams of calorie-providing foods, especially total carbohydrates and fats.

The percent Daily Value figures can be a little confusing to some consumers, because not all values represent targets to reach; some values represent thresholds to stay under. Nutritionists currently believe consuming too much sodium, for example, is associated with high blood pressure; too much added sugar may lead to increased risk of developing obesity and/or type 2 diabetes. Many people are trying to limit their intake of saturated fat and trans fat. In addition, people with very high blood cholesterol may need to limit dietary cholesterol. People with diabetes could be trying to limit total carbohydrates. People with kidney disease may have been told to limit protein. And while most Daily Values apply similarly to adult men and women, an exception is iron. The Daily Value for iron (18 mg per day) comes from the recommended intake for women of childbearing age, who need more iron because of the blood loss that occurs during the menstrual cycle. The recommended intake for men and non-menstruating women is actually only 8 mg per day. (See Question 25.)

10. How is serving size determined?

The serving sizes used on food labels are standardized for each type of food by the U.S. Food and Drug Administration (FDA) and reflect portions customarily consumed at one sitting. Standardized serving sizes allow consumers to easily compare products. However, the term "serving size" on food labels does not necessarily reflect other systems that use the term "serving size," such as the U.S. Department of Agriculture's MyPlate guidelines or the American Diabetes Association's Exchange Diet system. The term "serving size" is not even a recommendation on how much of a labeled food is best to eat. Individuals vary greatly in how many calories they need per day, so actual portion sizes of a given food consumed at a meal vary (and should vary) from person to person.

Because "serving size" is a rather vague term, the FDA uses the term "Reference Amounts Customarily Consumed" (RACC) in its literature for food manufacturers and publishes a table for food producers to consult when they are creating labels. (There are actually two sets of RACC tables: one for adults and children four years old and older; and one for infants and children under age four.) In this way, every label for tuna fish, for example, uses the same serving size. The FDA tables give the mandated serving size amounts in both household units and grams, and the manufacturer must figure out what represents a serving size for its product. The RACC tables also prescribe how the serving size is to be described on the label.

For example, if a food producer is trying to figure out the serving size for dried cranberries, it would check the RACC table, and find that the serving size for dried fruit is 40 g. Therefore, the Daily Values for the product would be based on a 40-g serving. To describe the serving size on the label, the producer would find the following serving size guideline for dried fruit in the RACC table:

___piece(s) (_ g) for large pieces (e.g., dates, figs, prunes); _ cup(s) (_ g) for small pieces (e.g., raisins)

Since dried cranberries are similar in size to raisins, the manufacturer would choose the second option. It would weigh out several 40-g servings and take the average size in terms of cups. The serving size on the package would read something like "serving size ¼ cup (40 g)."

Research shows that portion sizes have steadily increased over the past several decades. Because the serving sizes used on labels are generally intended to reflect the portion size a majority of people actually consume, they were updated by the FDA in 2016. Most serving size standards that changed were increased. For example, the serving size for ice cream increased from ½ cup to ⅔ cup. However, a few serving sizes decreased. These changes reflected current packaging customs. This explains why yogurt serving size decreased from 8 oz to 6 oz—because individually packaged yogurt products are most likely to be 6 oz.

Research has also shown that people consuming food from packages a little larger than one serving tend to eat the entire package. An interesting example is canned soup. The RACC for canned soup is only 245 g, or about 8.5 oz. But many cans of soup are around 14 or 15 oz, and surveys found that a majority of people consume the entire can's contents at one sitting. The 2016 labeling requirements reflect this knowledge and dictate that soup products of this larger size simply label the product as one serving, and provide % Daily Values for the entire can.

One of the most significant 2016 changes in the food labeling requirements concerns food packages that are technically more than one serving but no larger than three servings. These packages must list % Daily Values in two columns: one for the RACC serving size and one for the entire package. Consumers are likely to see this on packages of snack foods. Consider potato chips. The RACC serving size is 1 oz. However, some packages are 2 or 3 oz, and it is not unusual for people to finish these off in one sitting. Therefore, packages of potato chips that contain over 1 oz and up to 3 oz must have the dual column format.

11. With over 40 nutrients needed in the human diet, why are only a few on the label, and how are these chosen?

Food labels must be fairly small to fit neatly onto a food package. In addition, simpler labels are easier to read and use. Research shows that when consumers are given labels containing too much information, they are simply confused. People misunderstand the information presented or don't even try to use the information available for making decisions about food purchases and consumption. Therefore, food labels, especially the Nutrition Facts panel, must strike a balance between supplying the most important nutrition information in a helpful manner and including all the information that might be desired by some consumers. Thus, there is only room on the label for information about the most important nutrients and other food components.

The U.S. Food and Drug Administration (FDA) is the group that decides which nutrients and other information should be included on the Nutrition Facts panel. To make these decisions, the FDA gathers information from several sources, including the following.

- Public health reports: The FDA consulted several landmark reports when deciding what information should appear in the 1990s Nutrition

Facts panel. These reports included "The Surgeon General's Report on Nutrition and Health," published by the U.S. Department of Health and Human Services in 1988, and the National Research Council's 1989 report, "Diet and Health: Implications for Reducing Chronic Disease Risk." The National Research Council is part of the National Academies of Sciences, Engineering, and Medicine (NASEM). These important documents represented expert opinion regarding nutrition and health at that time. Additional reports over the past several decades continue to shape the work of the FDA.

- National public health goals: These goals are outlined in an important document called Healthy People 2020. (Health People 2030 is in development.) This document is produced by a large number of organizations, including the National Institutes of Health, the Centers for Disease Control and Prevention, and the U.S. Department of Agriculture. The Healthy People goals include reducing obesity rates and promoting positive health behaviors. Specific nutrition objectives include increasing consumption of fruits, vegetables, and whole grains; reducing consumption of saturated and trans fats; reducing consumption of added sugars and sodium; and increasing consumption of calcium.

- Food and Nutrition Board of the NASEM: This group of experts sets the Dietary Reference Intakes and studies other important public health issues. In the early 1990s, following the passage of the Nutrition Labeling and Education Act by Congress, NASEM formed a committee to study how food labels could be improved to help people improve their diets. This resulted in a report, entitled "Nutrition Labeling: Issues and Directions for the 1990s," that helped to guide the FDA in designing the 1990s Nutrition Facts panel. More recently, work by NASEM helped the FDA update the Daily Values used on food labels.

- Current peer-reviewed research reports: The FDA follows the current research on nutrition and health that is published in scientific journals.

- FDA-sponsored research: The FDA has worked with various scientific and industry groups to test different label formats. For example, different label formats have been shown to a variety of focus groups to determine potential consumer response. This type of research found that in general, people have a better understanding of numerical representation of percent Daily Value (e.g., 10% DV) than representations in graph form, for example, pie charts.

To sum up, the FDA chooses the nutrients required on the Nutrition Facts panel and other label elements, attempting to keep its work in line with national public health efforts. It is important that the messages people receive regarding diet and health are consistent, simple, and clear.

Why do some foods list % Daily Value for other nutrients in addition to those required on the Nutrition Facts panel?

The FDA permits food producers to voluntarily include information on a variety of nutrients; however, if a food label claims to have a significant amount of a given voluntary nutrient, the label must then supply information about how much of that nutrient is found in a serving, and the % Daily Value that the amount represents. Food producers may choose to do this to increase the appeal of their product.

The FDA prescribes that nutrients and other food components be listed in the following order. Voluntary components are indicated with a "V."

Calories
Calories from saturated fat—V
Total fat
Saturated fat
Trans fat
Polyunsaturated fat—V
Monounsaturated fat—V
Cholesterol
Sodium
Fluoride—V
Total carbohydrate
Dietary fiber
Soluble fiber—V
Insoluble fiber—V
Total sugars
Added sugars
Sugar alcohols—V
Protein
Vitamin D
Calcium
Iron
Potassium

The following nutrients are all voluntary and may be listed as desired or as required by a nutrient statement on the food package:

Vitamin A
Vitamin C
Vitamin E
Vitamin K
Thiamin
Riboflavin
Niacin
Vitamin B$_6$
Folate
Vitamin B$_{12}$
Biotin
Pantothenic acid
Phosphorus
Iodine
Magnesium
Zinc
Selenium
Copper
Manganese
Chromium
Molybdenum
Chloride
Choline

12. What are calories, and why are calories important on the Nutrition Facts panel?

On the Nutrition Facts panel, calories are used as a measure of the energy contained in food. Animals obtain energy for life processes by breaking down certain chemical bonds in food, in particular, the chemical bonds found in the macronutrients carbohydrates, proteins, and fats (and alcohol).

Scientists define a calorie as the amount of energy needed to raise the temperature of 1 g of water by 1°C under standard conditions. The calories on food labels are actually kilocalories. One kilocalorie equals 1,000 calories, or the amount of heat needed to raise the temperature of 1 kg of water by 1°C. This larger unit is used when discussing energy consumption and energy expenditure of larger animals such as humans. The term "Calorie," written with an initial capital letter, is also used to represent kilocalorie. However, in common language, the term "calorie" is often used simply as a general term for energy intake (from foods and beverages) and energy expenditure (as in "burning" calories during exercise).

The calorie first came into use as a unit of heat energy in early 19th-century France. In 1887 it was popularized in the United States by W. O. Atwater, when he began using the unit in his articles on food and in his tables of food composition. At the start of the 20th century, the word became further entrenched in common usage in the United States, due in great part to the U.S. Department of Agriculture (USDA) *Farmers' Bulletins* food databases. These were the first commonly available publications to list the calorie content of foods commonly consumed. As Americans became increasingly interested in weight management, the word began appearing in articles and books, garnering the interest of the lay public across the country.

The United States continues to use the term calorie on food labels, unlike most other countries that use kilojoules rather than kilocalories in describing food energy content. Most nations officially transitioned from the use of the calorie to use of the joule in 1954, when the International System of Units (SI) was adopted. Within the SI system, the unit for energy in any form is the joule (J), which corresponds with energy measurements and conversion factors in all other SI-based branches of science. One calorie equals 4.184 joules. Regardless of its context within the realm of international scientific standards, however, the calorie remains the primary unit of food energy for U.S. consumers.

Calories are important on labels because many people are interested in tracking and manipulating energy balance—adjusting the relationship between the energy they consume and the energy they expend. For example, people trying to lose weight should consume fewer calories than they expend so that they stimulate the use of stored energy, to reduce fat stores. Public health professionals have been concerned with increasing rates of obesity and obesity-related illness, and have advocated for making calorie figures more prominent on food labels so that consumers could readily find them. Thus, the newer food label features the word "Calories" and the calorie count in a larger font size than the older food label.

How accurate are these calorie figures?

The calorie number on the food label may not be entirely accurate for a few reasons. The Food and Drug Administration permits food manufacturers to calculate the calories in their food product in two different ways. The first way is known as the Atwater system. The manufacturer must determine the amounts of energy-containing compounds—carbohydrate, fat, and protein—in the food. Calories are calculated from these results. On average, carbohydrates and proteins deliver 4 kcal per gram, while fats deliver 9 kcal per gram. Calories contributed by dietary fiber are subtracted from the total to estimate actual calorie availability. However, errors occur because these general values do not always represent the exact bond energy available in a given food.

The process of rounding values for nutrient grams can also produce small errors in calorie content. Consumers sometimes notice that the calorie count does not appear to match the calories they calculate from the macronutrients. Grams of carbohydrate, protein, and fat are rounded to the nearest unit. For example, a food with 12.6 g would be rounded to 13 g. One with 0.4 g of carbohydrate would say "0 g" on the label. In fact, it is possible to have a "0 calorie" food that actually has a very small number of calories.

The second way manufacturers may calculate the calories in their food product is to use standard food composition tables from the USDA, calculating calories (and nutrition values) for their product based on product ingredients. Error can arise from differences between table values and the actual values for the ingredients used. Consider tomato sauce for example. The values given in the USDA table for tomatoes may be slightly different from those of the actual tomatoes used by the manufacturer.

Another potential source of inaccuracy occurs because people do not necessarily digest and absorb all of the bond energy contained in a food. Atwater and the USDA estimated the energy contained in a food's chemical bonds with an instrument known as a calorimeter. This device functions by completely burning a given food sample in a chamber that is surrounded by a fluid, such as water. The temperature change of the fluid reflects the energy value of the food. Temperature change then can be directly converted into calories. People obtain energy from the chemical bonds in foods in a very different way: digestion and absorption. There are many steps in these processes, and many things can happen to enhance or obstruct these processes along the way. For example, foods that are already highly processed are more easily and quickly digested and absorbed. The health of the gastrointestinal tract influences digestion and absorption. The types of bacteria living in the large intestine also appear to influence energy availability.

It is interesting to compare the absorption of similar foods in processed versus less-processed states to see the difference between theoretical calorie content and the actual number of calories absorbed by average people. Less-processed foods, especially those higher in fiber and certain types of starches that are difficult for the body to break down (resistant starches), may actually provide fewer calories than shown on the food label. For example, compare peanut butter to peanuts. According to a 2008 research study by Dr. C. J. Traoret and colleagues, most of the calories found in peanut butter, peanut flour, and peanut oil were absorbed after consumption by human volunteers, but about 38% of the calories in unprocessed peanuts were not absorbed. Cooking has effects similar to processing, increasing calorie availability. The results of such studies suggest that calorie counts on the labels of processed foods are probably closer to the actual number of calories absorbed by most people from those foods.

How much do these errors in calorie counts really matter? The calorie figures on the Nutrition Facts panel are still a useful guideline in many ways. They help consumers compare food products and provide at least a general guideline regarding the energy provided by the given food product.

13. What is meant by total fat, and why is total fat listed on the Nutrition Facts panel?

Total fat, as the name implies, represents the fat content, including all types of fats, in a serving of a food product. Fat refers to both oils and solid fats in the diet. Oils are liquid at room temperature, while solid fats, like butter or the fat in meat, are solid. Fat is one of the three macronutrients used by the body to make energy. Fat is a particularly concentrated source of energy, contributing 9 kcal per gram, while proteins and carbohydrates contribute 4 kcal per gram.

The primary components of fat in the diet are structures called fatty acids. Fatty acids are organic compounds composed of hydrocarbon chains with an organic acid (carboxyl) group at one end and a methyl (CH_3) group at the other end. Fatty acids are found not only in foods but also in the body.

There are many types of fatty acids, and their function in the body varies with their structure. Many fatty acids, such as the long-chain polyunsaturated fatty acids (PUFAs), are beneficial to health. Ingestion of large amounts of saturated fatty acids from animal products is thought to increase risk of artery disease, the most common type of cardiovascular disease. The body is able to manufacture some types of fatty acids from fat, carbohydrate, and protein in the diet. However, some types of fatty acids must come from the diet. These are called essential fatty acids, and they include alpha-linolenic acid (ALA) and linoleic acid.

Fatty acids vary in the length of their hydrocarbon chains and in the types of bonds between the carbon atoms in these chains. Fatty acids found in foods usually have an even number of carbons, with a chain length of 4–24 carbons. Fatty acids with a chain length of fewer than six carbons are called short-chain fatty acids; medium-chain and long-chain fatty acids have 6–10, and 12 or more carbons, respectively. Some nutritionists use the term "very long-chain fatty acids" to refer to fatty acids with 20 or more carbons.

The carbon atoms in the fatty acid hydrocarbon chain may form single or double bonds with each other. Saturated fatty acids refer to fatty acids in which the bonds between carbon atoms are all single. Single carbon-carbon bonds are more stable than double bonds and affect the behavior of these fatty acids. For example, saturated fats tend to be more stable at higher temperatures. This explains why butter (higher in saturated fatty acids) is a solid at room temperature, while plant oils are not (lower in saturated fatty acids).

Unsaturated fatty acids have at least one carbon-carbon double bond. Monounsaturated fatty acids have one carbon-carbon double bond, while PUFAs have more than one. The location of this carbon-carbon double bond helps to name the fatty acid and affects the fatty acid's structure and behavior in the body. Omega-3 fatty acids have the carbon-carbon double bond at the third carbon from the methyl end of the fatty acid. Dietary sources of omega-3 fatty acids include fish oils and some plant and nut oils. Fish oils contain special long-chain omega-3 fatty acids, including docosahexaenoic acid (DHA) and eicosapentaenoic acid (EPA). DHA and EPA are associated with beneficial health effects, including reduced levels of inflammation and slower rates of blood clotting. This is why many public health recommendations suggest that people increase their consumption of fish. Oily fish such as salmon, tuna, sardines, mackerel, and herring have the highest concentrations of these fatty acids. ALA is another type of omega-3 fatty acid, although its effects on the health variables mentioned earlier do not appear to be as strong as those of DHA and EPA. On the other hand, omega-6 fatty acids, found primarily in plant oils, are associated with higher levels of inflammation and increased rates of blood clotting.

Trans fatty acids (trans fats) are usually created by hydrogenation, a process used by food product manufacturers to make fatty acids in foods more saturated, thus more stable and with a longer shelf life. While trans fats technically have a carbon-carbon double bond, the arrangement of other atoms around the bond leads to a shape of the fatty acid that is more similar to saturated fatty acids. Greater intake of trans fats in the diet has been linked to higher rates of artery disease. Trans fats may increase this risk through effects on blood lipid levels (raising LDL ("bad") cholesterol levels and lowering HDL ("good") cholesterol levels), the function of the artery lining, and making the blood more likely to form blood clots.

The amount of total fat in a serving of a food product is included on the Nutrition Facts panel because many consumers are interested in knowing how much fat is in their diet. Eating plans often suggest some sort of ratio for carbohydrate, protein, and fat calories in the diet, so food labels give consumers the information needed for these calculations. Other eating plans may prescribe a limit for the number of fat grams ingested per day. In addition to listing the amount of total fat in a food product, the Nutrition Facts panel supplies information on how much saturated fat (listed as sat fat) and trans fat is found in a serving of the labeled product. (See questions 14 and 15.)

The Nutrition Facts panel also provides a percent Daily Value figure for total fat. This value is based on the amount of fat considered to be healthy for people consuming 2,000 kcal/day. The Daily Value for total fat is 65 g. This value is drawn from the Acceptable Macronutrient Distribution Range (AMDR) recommendations from the Food and Nutrition Board of the National Academies of Science, Engineering, and Medicine (NASEM). NASEM recommends that healthy adults consume about 20% to 35% of their daily calories as fat. For people consuming 2,000 kcal/day, this would mean 400 to 700 kcal of fat, or about 44 to 78 g of fat. (Fat supplies 9 kcal/g.) The Daily Value of 65 g is close to the middle of this very broad range.

Extensive discussion concerning recommendations regarding total fat intake continues in the nutrition field. In general, the focus has been shifting away from limiting total fat intake to limiting saturated and trans fats. While for decades the U.S. Department of Agriculture's Dietary Guidelines for Americans had urged consumers to reduce intake of total fats, the 2015–2020 Dietary Guidelines for Americans no longer recommends limiting overall fat intake. Instead, the Guidelines, reflecting the recommendations of many professional health groups, urge consumers to choose sources of fat higher in unsaturated fats, and to limit intake of saturated and trans fats.

An illustration of this shift can be found in one of the differences between the previous and the current Nutrition Facts labels. The previous label listed "calories from fat" next to the calories figure. "Calories from fat" is no longer included on the current Nutrition Facts label.

Evidence of this change in focus regarding fat is also apparent in the Food and Drug Administration (FDA) regulation of the word "healthy" on food labels. Until recently, a food labeled as "healthy" was required to be low in total fat content. Beginning in 2016, the FDA stopped requiring a product using the word "healthy" on its label to be low in total fat. Instead, the FDA declared that to use the word "healthy," the majority (over 50%) of the fat content of the product must be composed of unsaturated fats. In addition, the amounts of monounsaturated and polyunsaturated fats must be stated on the label.

The FDA regulates several fat-related nutrient content claims. The most common include the following:

"Light or lite"—This qualifier may be used on food products that meet the definition for "low fat" or "low calorie."

- The term must explain the use of the word light, for example, "light—low in fat."
- In addition, fat content must be reduced by at least 50% per serving, compared to a "reference" product. For example, the term "light" may be used for potato chips that are lower in fat than ordinary potato chips.

"Fat-free"—Foods with this label must have fewer than 0.5 g of fat per serving. In addition, they may not include an ingredient containing significant amounts of fat, for example, oil or nuts.

"Low-fat"—These foods must have 3 or fewer grams of fat per serving.

"Reduced fat or less fat"—Foods with this label must have at least 25% less fat per serving compared to a suitable reference food.

On labels for meat, "lean" indicates that the meat has less than 10 g of total fat, 4.5 g or less of saturated fat, and less than 95 mg of cholesterol per 100 g of meat. "Extra lean" means that the meat has less than 5 g of total fat, less than 2 g of saturated fat, and less than 95 mg of cholesterol.

14. What is saturated fat, and why is a food's saturated fat content included on the Nutrition Facts panel?

The terms "saturated fat" and "sat fat" are abbreviations for saturated fatty acids. Fatty acids are the most common component of fat in the diet. Fatty acids are chains with a backbone of carbon atoms connected to one another, with hydrogen molecules bonded to the carbons. (See question 13.)

The carbon atoms in the fatty acid hydrocarbon chain may form single or double bonds with each other. Saturated fatty acids refer to fatty acids in which the bonds between carbon atoms are all single. Saturated fatty acids are "saturated" with hydrogens; that is, the carbon chain binds as many hydrogens as possible to each carbon in the chain. Saturated fats are most plentiful in fats that are solid at room temperature, such as meat fat, butter, palm oil, and coconut oil.

The amount of saturated fat in a serving of a food is included on the Nutrition Facts panel because higher levels of saturated fat intake are associated with increased risk of artery disease, the leading cause of heart disease and stroke. Many consumers have experienced significant confusion regarding dietary saturated fat recommendations, as a number of nutrition sources have questioned the strength of the link between saturated fat intake and heart disease risk. Headlines such as "Butter is back" have frequently graced the pages of scientific and lay publications. Part of the confusion stems from the fact that it is difficult to look at one dietary component, such as saturated fat, without consideration for the daily food intake pattern. For example, a diet that is relatively high in saturated fat is often also high in red and processed meat and lower in plant foods and helpful plant chemicals such as dietary fiber and antioxidants. The 2015–2020 U.S. Dietary Guidelines emphasize the development of an overall healthy eating pattern for this reason, rather than concentrating too much on individual food components.

Complicating the saturated fatty acid relationship to health even further is the fact that there are several types of saturated fatty acids in the human diet. Fatty acids vary in their metabolic effects depending not only on their degree of saturation but also upon the length of their carbon chains. The most common saturated fatty acids in the human diet have an even number of 4–20 carbons in their chains. For example, butyric acid, a saturated fat plentiful in dairy fat, contains only four carbons in its chain. Lauric acid contains 12 carbons and stearic acid 18. Food label readers may have observed that food products made from coconut fat are high in saturated fat. Yet coconut oil products have become popular among some consumers because proponents of these products claim that the high percentage of medium chain fatty acids (fatty acids with 6–12 carbons) is healthful rather than harmful, although sound evidence for this statement is lacking.

At this time, the most respected advice concerning saturated fatty intake is that most people would benefit from replacing foods high in saturated fats with foods high in monounsaturated and polyunsaturated fats. Healthful foods high in unsaturated fats include seafood; nuts; mayonnaise; salad dressings; and plant oils such as olive, canola, and soy oils.

The Nutrition Facts panel gives information about the amount of saturated fat per serving both in grams and as a percent of Daily Value. The Daily Value for saturated fat is 20 g/day. This is based on the National Academies of Science, Engineering, and Medicine recommendation that calories from saturated fat comprise no more than 10% of the calories in the diet. For a calorie intake of 2,000 kcal/day, this would be the equivalent of 200 kcal, or 22 g of saturated fat. (Each gram of any kind of fat, including saturated fat, contains 9 kcal.)

A food label may make the following claims: "low in saturated fat," "low saturated fat," "contains a small amount of saturated fat," "low source of saturated fat," or "a little saturated fat" if the product contains less than 1 g of saturated fat per serving, and if less than 15% of the calories in the food come from saturated fats. If the food product qualifies for this description without the need for special processing or reformulation to lower saturated fat content, it must be labeled to indicate that low in saturated fat is typical of all brands of that food. For example, if the label is advertising that raspberries are a food low in saturated fat, it would state, for example, "raspberries, a low saturated fat food."

A food label may claim "saturated fat free," "free of saturated fat," "no saturated fat," "zero saturated fat," "without saturated fat," "trivial sources of saturated fat," "negligible source of saturated fat," or "dietarily insignificant source of saturated fat" if it contains less than 0.5 g of saturated fat per serving. However, the product must also contain less than 0.5 g of trans fatty acids per serving. In addition, the label must state the amount of cholesterol if cholesterol content is 2 mg or more per serving, and the amount of total fat if total fat content is 0.5 g or more per serving.

The terms "reduced saturated fat," "reduced in saturated fat," "saturated fat reduced," "less saturated fat," "lower saturated fat," or "lower in saturated fat" must explain how the food compares to a standard and similar reference product. The reduced saturated fat food must contain at least 25% less saturated fat per serving than an appropriate reference food, and the label must explain the details of this comparison. The label must say, for example, "reduced saturated fat. Contains 50 % less saturated fat than our regular macaroni and cheese." Labels should also explain how the quantities of saturate fat differ between the two foods, for example, "Saturated fat content has been reduced from 3 g per 3 oz to 2 g per 3 oz." Reduced saturated fat claims may not be made for foods already labeled "low saturated fat."

15. What is trans fat, and why is trans fat content listed on the Nutrition Facts panel?

Trans fatty acids (trans fats) are a type of fatty acid (a common type of fat in the diet) that occurs both in nature and as a result of the hydrogenation of vegetable oils. Most of the trans fats in the human diet come from food products containing hydrogenated or partially hydrogenated oils. Foods that typically use these oils include crackers, cookies, doughnuts, and baked goods such as pastries.

Hydrogenation is a process used by food product manufacturers to make fatty acids in foods more saturated, and thus more stable at room temperature. This stability gives food products a longer shelf life. Foods with unsaturated oils as ingredients can develop a rancid smell and taste as the carbon-carbon double bonds in these fats are vulnerable to oxidation.

Most carbon-carbon double bonds in plant oils are found in what is called a cis formation. A cis formation means that the hydrogens attached to the carbons forming the double bond are on the same side of that double bond, which causes a bend in the hydrocarbon chain. During the process of hydrogenation, hydrogen is added to vegetable oils. In this process most of the carbon-carbon double bonds in the unsaturated fats are transformed to single bonds, as the carbons pick up additional hydrogen atoms. But sometimes the process is incomplete, and the carbon-carbon double bonds remain. Trans fats result when the hydrogens of this bond undergo rearrangement and end up on opposite sides of the double bond, a formation known as a trans formation. It is not a goal of hydrogenation to produce trans fats; these are simply a by-product of this process. The trans formation removes the bend typically found in the cis formation, which makes the fatty acid hydrocarbon chain straighter, and structurally similar to a saturated fatty acid. (A saturated fatty acid has no carbon-carbon double bonds.)

The amount of trans fat in a serving of a food product is listed on the product's Nutrition Facts panel because research suggests that people whose diets are high in trans fats have a greater risk of cardiovascular disease. Researchers do not know exactly why a higher intake of trans fats is associated with greater risk of artery disease. Trans fats do appear to increase blood levels of low-density lipoprotein cholesterol (often known as the "bad" cholesterol) and decrease blood levels of high-density lipoprotein cholesterol (often known as the "good" cholesterol). These changes are associated with increased development of arterial plaque and cardiovascular disease. A high intake of trans fat is also associated with more arterial inflammation, which alters the health and function of the arterial lining (the endothelium) and increases the tendency of the blood to form clots inside the arteries.

In 2015, the Food and Drug Administration (FDA) removed trans fats from the list of food components generally recognized as safe, so trans fats are no longer permitted to be added to foods. Researchers believe this could prevent thousands of heart attacks each year. This ruling does not affect the very small amounts of trans fats naturally found in some meat and dairy products. New food products designed after June 18, 2018, could not add hydrogenated or partially hydrogenated oils to their products. Other food products were required to stop using hydrogenated and partially hydrogenated oils by January 1, 2020. A food company can petition the FDA for permission to use partially hydrogenated oils with small amounts of trans fats if the company submits studies showing the use of the oil is safe.

The FDA has ruled that food products need not declare "0 g" of trans fat on the Nutrition Facts panel if that food contains less than 0.5 g of total fat in a serving, and if no claims are stated on the label about fat, fatty acid, or cholesterol content. The statement "not a significant source of trans fat" may be placed at the bottom of the Nutrition Facts panel.

The Nutrition Facts panel does not list a percent Daily Value for trans fats, since the FDA, following the lead of scientific advisers, declares there is not a safe level of consumption. The National Academies of Science, Engineering, and Medicine recommend that "trans fat consumption be as low as possible while consuming a nutritionally adequate diet."

Some consumers are concerned that the FDA permits companies to label trans fat amounts as 0 g on the Nutrition Facts panel as long as trans fat amounts are less than 0.5 g per serving. This means that theoretically, people who eat a lot of products with hydrogenated vegetable oils could potentially consume significant amounts of trans fats, even though the Nutrition Facts panels of the foods consumed state that the products contain 0 g of trans fats per serving. Consumers can find out if they are consuming hydrogenated oils by reading a product's ingredient list. Any item with the term "hydrogenated" or "partially hydrogenated" in it may contribute a small amount of trans fat to the food product.

16. What is cholesterol, and why is cholesterol content included on the Nutrition Facts panel?

Cholesterol belongs to a group of chemical compounds called sterols. Cholesterol is found both in foods and in the body. Cholesterol is made from four linked hydrocarbon rings with a hydrocarbon group at one end and a hydroxyl group at the other end. It is an important membrane lipid, supporting cell membrane permeability (regulating how easily important molecules cross the cell membrane) and membrane structural fluidity. Cholesterol is found in varying degrees in practically all animal cell membranes. The body manufactures steroid hormones such as progesterone, testosterone, estrogens, and cortisol from cholesterol. Cholesterol is also the precursor of vitamin D. The liver manufactures bile from cholesterol. Bile is important for the digestion and absorption of fats and fat-soluble vitamins. Cholesterol can be obtained from animal products in the diet, but most of it, around 85% in omnivores, is synthesized by the body. People who do not consume animal products easily produce all of the cholesterol they need. The liver is the major site of cholesterol synthesis, but the small intestine also produces significant amounts of cholesterol. The rate of synthesis of cholesterol by the body can vary greatly, based on several factors, including how much cholesterol is consumed in the diet. Blood levels of cholesterol and cholesterol-transport compounds are somewhat predictive of a person's risk for the development of artery disease and its complications, including heart attack and stroke. Overall diet pattern, as well as several dietary components, appears to influence blood cholesterol levels.

The Nutrition Facts panel includes a food's cholesterol content because of a long history of research into the association of dietary cholesterol with blood cholesterol levels. Cholesterol in both the diet and as a component of artery disease came under scrutiny in the 1950s as researchers began to investigate artery disease etiology. Artery disease is marked by the development of deposits, called plaques, in the artery lining, causing a swelling and thickening of the lining, and sometimes rupture of the plaques. Observing that arterial plaque contains high concentrations of cholesterol and other lipids, researchers began to explore the association between dietary cholesterol and fats, blood cholesterol levels, artery disease development and progression, and endpoints such as heart attack and stroke. Researchers originally proposed that high amounts of cholesterol in the diet would be linked to high amounts of cholesterol in the arteries, but this does not appear to be the case. Experts now believe that intake of dietary fat and cholesterol does influence artery disease development, but in complex ways, primarily through the behavior of cholesterol-carrying compounds known as lipoproteins.

Cholesterol is transported from its sites of synthesis or absorption to the sites of use, and finally to the liver for excretion by transport molecules called lipoproteins. Lipoproteins are composed of cholesterol, triglycerides, phospholipids, and proteins. They have nonpolar, hydrophobic regions in the center, with polar regions on the exterior, allowing the compounds to travel in the aqueous environment of the body. Lipoproteins exist in several forms. They are classified based on their composition, which influences their relative weight or density. Higher levels of low-density lipoprotein (LDL) cholesterol are associated with increased risk of artery disease. LDLs appear to promote arterial damage when they become oxidized and bind with the artery lining. Higher levels of high-density lipoprotein (HDL) cholesterol are associated with lower risk of artery disease. LDLs are known as the "bad" cholesterol. HDLs are known as the "good" cholesterol because they transport cholesterol from plasma and deliver it to the liver where cholesterol is converted into bile and other products, and excreted.

High serum LDL cholesterol levels increase artery disease risk. This risk was first observed in people with abnormally high serum cholesterol levels because of an inherited condition known as familial hypercholesterolemia. This condition is characterized by deposition of cholesterol in various tissues. Familial hypercholesterolemia is not due to excess dietary cholesterol, but to the inability to remove LDL cholesterol from the blood. Familial hypercholesterolemia is associated with an increased risk of early artery disease, and a higher risk of cardiovascular disease, including heart attack and stroke.

As research continued to accumulate evidence that blood levels of total cholesterol, LDL cholesterol, and HDL cholesterol are related to artery disease risk, the U.S. National Heart, Lung, and Blood Institute launched the National Cholesterol Education Program in 1985. The program has promoted public education regarding the importance of diagnosing and treating high cholesterol levels. High LDL cholesterol levels can be reduced by both lifestyle measures and medications. Lifestyle measures that promote healthful blood cholesterol levels include regular physical activity, weight control to achieve healthful body fat levels, and a heart-healthy diet.

Does dietary cholesterol actually influence blood cholesterol levels?

After decades of research on the dietary cholesterol–blood cholesterol relationship, scientists no longer believe that the relationship is very direct or strong, and that evidence is not available for stating a quantitative limit for dietary cholesterol. Cholesterol synthesis, transport, metabolism, and absorption from the small intestine are complex and influenced by many variables. In fact, while the 2015 U.S. Dietary Guidelines advocated limiting cholesterol intake, they no longer highlighted a numerical suggested limit for consumption as they had in the past. Previous versions of the U.S. Dietary Guidelines had advocated consuming less than 100 mg of dietary cholesterol per 1,000 kcals of food intake per day. For most consumers, this translated into an intake of less than 200–300 mg/day.

Studies on blood cholesterol, foods, and diet pattern have found that dietary change is sometimes helpful for slightly reducing blood LDL-cholesterol levels, especially for people whose blood cholesterol level is slightly high but not high enough to qualify for the prescription of cholesterol-lowering medication. Dietary patterns associated with improved blood cholesterol levels include almost any weight loss diet, including low-carbohydrate diets (e.g., the Atkins diet), low-fat diets, and Mediterranean-type diets. Weight-loss diets are effective for short-term cholesterol reduction. For long-term weight-loss maintenance and blood cholesterol control, both low-fat and Mediterranean-type diets have good support. Nutrition professionals recommend diets high in plant foods, including fruits, vegetables, and legumes. Consumption of foods high in saturated fats and cholesterol, such as high-fat meats, processed meats, should be reduced. While intake of dietary cholesterol does not appear to have a strong effect on serum cholesterol levels in healthy people, most public health organizations note that many foods high in cholesterol can also be high in saturated fat, and many health professionals continue to recommend keeping daily cholesterol intake below 300 mg per day, the current Daily Value used on food labels. People with type 2 diabetes, obesity, or heart disease appear to be most sensitive to cholesterol intake and may benefit from limiting consumption of foods that are high in cholesterol.

17. What is sodium, and why is sodium content listed on the Nutrition Facts panel?

Sodium is an essential nutrient, a mineral found primarily in salts. Salts are ionic compounds that result from the combining of an acid and a base.

Table salt is a combination of the positively and negatively charged ions sodium and chloride. In an aqueous environment, such as that in the body, sodium chloride dissolves to produce the positively charged ion, or electrolyte, sodium, and the negatively charged chloride. Table salt is the primary source of sodium in the diet, and the terms "salt" and "sodium" are often used interchangeably when discussing dietary recommendations.

Sodium performs many essential functions in the body. It is an important electrolyte in fluids found outside of body cells. It is found in the fluid that surrounds body cells (interstitial fluid) and in blood plasma (the liquid portion of blood in which blood cells are suspended). It works with other major electrolytes, including chloride and potassium, to regulate the distribution of water throughout the body. Sodium is essential for nerve conduction and muscle contraction, processes that rely on the electrochemical gradient maintained on either side of cell membranes. Special ion pumps embedded in cell membranes maintain this electrochemical difference by regulating the concentration of ions in these two regions. The concentration of sodium is about 10 times higher outside of the cell than inside of the cell; the concentration of potassium is about 30 times higher inside cells. The activity of these ion pumps accounts for a significant portion of the energy expended as part of a person's resting metabolic rate.

Sodium absorption in the gastrointestinal tract enhances the absorption of other nutrients, including amino acids and glucose. Sodium concentration in the plasma influences the activity of the hormones that in turn influence the kidney's regulation of water balance, blood volume, and blood pressure.

Sodium content is listed on the Nutrition Facts panel because, unlike most other minerals needed in the diet, sodium is more commonly associated with health problems rather than health benefits. People enjoy the taste of salt, and salt is used as a flavor enhancer and preservative in many foods. Salt is widely available and consumed at levels significantly above the recommended minimum in countries around the world.

The most common health problem associated with excess dietary sodium is hypertension (high blood pressure). Hypertension contributes to both heart disease and stroke, leading causes of death in North America and around the world. A high sodium intake may also contribute to osteoporosis and kidney stones. People with certain health problems, especially hypertension, heart failure, diabetes, and kidney disease, are advised to limit sodium intake to very low levels. Reading food labels to regulate sodium intake is an important part of disease prevention and management for many people.

Sodium deficiency, or hyponatremia, is relatively rare. It is diagnosed by low blood sodium levels. Hyponatremia is usually caused by dehydration accompanying illness, use of diuretics, or kidney disease. It can also be caused by excessive intake of water, sometimes combined with impaired fluid excretion, occurring most commonly in people engaged in prolonged exercise events. Symptoms of hyponatremia include nausea, vomiting, muscle cramps, headaches, fatigue, and disorientation. Without intervention, hyponatremia can lead to brain damage, seizures, coma, and death.

The Daily Value for sodium is less than 2,400 mg. However, the Dietary Reference Intake for adults is 2,300 mg/day. People with hypertension, heart failure, diabetes, and kidney disease are often advised to consume even less. Experts continue to debate exactly how low sodium intakes should go, and at what intake level health problems become more likely to develop. Research suggests that a high intake of other important electrolytes, such as potassium, magnesium, and calcium, may blunt the negative effect of sodium.

People in the United States currently consume on average about 3,400 mg/day of sodium. A majority of this, approximately 75%, comes from prepared/packaged foods and restaurant meals. Interestingly, only about 5% of the sodium in the U.S. diet is added by consumers at the table as they salt their food. About 6% comes from meals prepared at home. And 14% of the sodium in the U.S. diet is naturally occurring in food. Dairy products such as milk and cheese are naturally high in sodium.

Since a majority of sodium in the diet derives from packaged foods and restaurant meals, public health efforts aimed at reducing sodium intake are often focused on encouraging or requiring food manufacturers to reduce sodium levels in their products. And health care providers urge patients needing to reduce sodium intake to make more of their meals at home, and to compare food labels for similar items when grocery shopping. The Food and Drug Administration (FDA) advises sodium-conscious consumers to check the %Daily Value (DV) figures for sodium on labels. Foods that provide 5 %DV or less for sodium are generally considered low in sodium, while foods containing 20 %DV or more for sodium are high in sodium.

Food manufacturers seek to take advantage of the large market of consumers shopping for food products with lower levels of sodium and have created hundreds of products designed to appeal to this group. The FDA regulates food label nutrient content claims for sodium. These claims can be somewhat confusing. Terms such as "sodium free," "low sodium," "reduced sodium," "light," and "healthy" all have special meaning with reference to sodium content per serving size and are described here.

"Sodium free"—These foods contain only a trivial amount of sodium per serving.

- These foods contain less than 5 mg per serving.
- They contain no ingredient that is sodium chloride or generally understood to contain sodium.
- Food labeled "salt free" must meet criterion for "sodium free."
- The words "no salt added" and "unsalted" are allowed if no salt is added during processing. However, the labels for these foods must declare "This is not a sodium-free food" on the information panel if the food is not "sodium free."

"Very low sodium"—These foods contain 35 mg or less per serving (or per 50 g if serving size is small); for meals and main dishes, 35 mg or less per 100 g.

"Low sodium"—These foods contain 140 mg or less per serving (or per 50 g if serving size is small); for meals and main dishes, 140 mg or less per 100g.

For "sodium free," "very low," or "low" claims, labels must indicate if food meets a definition without benefit of special processing, alteration, formulation, or reformulation. When sodium content is reduced through processing, then the claims "reduced sodium" or "light (lite) in sodium" must be used. The definitions for these terms follow.

"Reduced sodium"—This term refers to foods in which the level of sodium is reduced by 25%. In other words, the food contains at least 25% less sodium per serving size than an appropriate reference food (or, for meals and main dishes, at least 25% less sodium per 100 g). The reference food may not be "low sodium." For sodium-reduced products, if sodium is reduced by 50% or more and the food does not meet the definition of "low calorie" or "low fat," the nutrient content claim must say "light in sodium." If sodium is reduced by 50% or more and the food meets the definition of "low calories" and "low fat," the claim "light" may be used without further qualification.

"Light" or "lite in sodium"—As noted earlier, in these products, sodium is reduced by at least 50% per serving size. For meals and main dishes, "light in sodium" must meet definition for "low in sodium."

"Lightly salted"—This term has a special meaning, that the food contains 50% less sodium than is normally added to the reference food. If the food does not meet the definition for "low sodium," it must state that on the information panel, that is, "not a low sodium food." This is important because shoppers might think that "lightly salted" is the same thing as a low sodium food. But lightly salted potato chips, for example, might still not be a low sodium food.

"Healthy"—An individual food labeled as "healthy" must meet certain criteria for several nutrients. For sodium, a food labeled as "healthy" must contain 480 mg or less per serving size. Foods with a serving size less than or equal to 30 g or 2 tablespoons must contain 480 mg or less per 50 g. A meal or main dish labeled as healthy must meet several criteria, including for sodium 600 mg or less per labeled serving.

18. What are carbohydrates, and why is carbohydrate content listed on the Nutrition Facts panel?

Carbohydrates are a large group of organic molecules that include sugars, starches, and most types of dietary fiber. The word "carbohydrate" comes from the raw materials from which carbohydrates are made. Plants make carbohydrates from carbon dioxide (source of the term "carbo") and water ("hydrate"), using energy from the sun. All carbohydrates contain only carbon, hydrogen, and oxygen. Plant carbohydrates provide energy and dietary fiber to the animals that eat them. Animals also produce carbohydrates from the food they eat, primarily for the purpose of storing energy. Informally, the term carbohydrate (or even "carbs") is used to refer to foods that contain relatively high concentrations of carbohydrate molecules. The human body can harness the energy stored in some carbohydrate structures to make energy. Most cultures of the world rely on foods high in carbohydrates for a majority of daily calories.

The simplest carbohydrate structures are called monosaccharides. Monosaccharides provide the basic units for other carbohydrate molecules. Typical dietary sugars are composed of two monosaccharides and are called disaccharides. Larger structures composed of many monosaccharide units are called oligosaccharides (3–10 units) and polysaccharides (more than 10 units).

Sugars, also known as simple carbohydrates, are relatively small molecules of carbohydrate found naturally in fruits and vegetables, as well as milk. They are especially concentrated in sweeteners such as table sugar (usually made from sugar beets or sugar cane), honey, molasses, and maple syrup. Corn syrup is a sweetener made from the sugar in corn. Many food products contain added sweeteners. Sugars are discussed more fully in Question 20.

Complex carbohydrates are larger molecules of carbohydrate and include starches and some types of dietary fibers. Oligosaccharides consist of 3–10 glucose units and are found in a variety of foods. Oligosaccharides can serve as starches or dietary fibers, depending on whether or not they can be broken down in the digestive tract. Common oligosaccharides include raffinose (three glucose units) and stachyose (four glucose units), found in legumes. Human digestive enzymes are unable to break the molecular bonds that hold the glucose units together, but intestinal bacteria are able to break these bonds, producing intestinal gas in the process. Human milk contains over 100 different oligosaccharides that help babies in a number of ways, including binding with pathogens, serving as food sources for helpful bacteria, and promoting normal infant brain development.

Polysaccharides contain more than 10 glucose units and are often composed of hundreds of glucose units strung together in various formations. These formations determine the properties of the starch, including the speed at which it is digested and absorbed (a quality known as glycemic index) and its behavior in recipes. The two primary starch formations in plants are amylose and amylopectin. Amylose is composed of long straight chains of glucose units. Amylopectin contains long branching chains of glucose units. Starch polysaccharides are found in plant foods and products made from plants. Grains and grain products; root vegetables such as potatoes, carrots, beets, and cassava; and vegetables that are the seeds of plants, such as corn, peas, and beans are high in starch. During digestion, starches are broken down into glucose units.

Glycogen is a form of starch manufactured by animals. However, glycogen is not present in significant amounts in the diet, since there is not much glycogen left in animal flesh after slaughtering. Humans make glycogen from carbohydrates in food. Glycogen is stored primarily in the liver and in skeletal muscles.

Dietary fiber refers to structures that are not broken down by the digestive system. Dietary fiber comes primarily from plants. Most types of dietary fiber, such as cellulose, are composed of carbohydrates. Humans lack the necessary digestive enzymes for breaking down these structures, so they pass through the digestive system, adding bulk to the stools. Adequate intake of dietary fiber contributes to good health. Most dietary guidelines encourage people to consume adequate amounts of vegetables, fruits, legumes, and whole grains to promote a healthy intake of dietary fiber.

The Dietary Reference Intake (DRI) for carbohydrates is at least 130 g/day for both children and adults. The DRI is based on the carbohydrate intake that will prevent the symptoms of low blood sugar, such as dizziness, nausea, confusion, and fatigue.

The Acceptable Macronutrient Distribution Range (AMDR) for carbohydrates is 45 to 65% of total energy (total kilocalories) consumed. One gram of nonfiber carbohydrate supplies about 4 kcal. Therefore, for a 2,000 kcal/day food intake, carbohydrate intake recommendations would be 225–325 g/day. For 2,500 kcal/day, it would be 281–406 g/day. Most North Americans consume at least 50% of their calories as carbohydrates, which amounts to over 250 g/day.

The Daily Value for carbohydrates used on the Nutrition Facts panel is 275 g/day. This value is based on a caloric intake of 2,000 kcal. The food label provides values for carbohydrate both in grams per serving, and as a percent DV. It is important to note that the 275 g/day figure is a rough guideline, neither an upper nor a lower limit, and most consumers will find the AMDR more helpful.

On the food label, "total carbohydrate" refers to all carbohydrates in the food product, including "dietary fiber" and "total sugars." The dietary fiber and total sugars contribute to the total carbohydrate figure. Total carbohydrate content is listed on the Nutrition Facts panel because many consumers are interested in knowing the total carbohydrate content of a food product, and of the carbohydrate content of their diet. These include people trying to lose weight who are on diets that limit or prescribe a specific carbohydrate intake. They also include people with diabetes or prediabetes, or a family history of diabetes. People trying to stay in ketosis and following a ketogenic diet strictly limit carbohydrate intake and must keep a careful track of carbohydrate ingestion. And athletes may be monitoring their carbohydrate intake in order to improve athletic performance.

People trying to lose weight often have a love/hate relationship with carbohydrates. Many people regard carbohydrate foods as "bad." Yet carbohydrates are contained within a wide range of foods. Some of these foods, such as most vegetables, are generally regarded as very nutritious. Other foods high in carbohydrates, such as cakes, cookies, and soft drinks, obtain a majority of their calories from processed grains and sugars, and are typically higher in empty calories (calories that deliver little nutritive value).

People with diabetes or prediabetes have difficulty absorbing glucose from the bloodstream into the cells of the body because of problems producing or using the hormone insulin. (Glucose enters the bloodstream either from the digestive system, after a meal, or when it is released from the liver.) People taking medications to regulate blood sugar may need to adjust medication dosage to complement carbohydrate intake, as well as other factors, such as physical activity, that affect blood glucose level.

A ketogenic diet severely limits carbohydrate intake so that a person is primarily metabolizing ketones, made by the body from fat, to produce energy. The body increases its manufacture of ketones when its supply of carbohydrate is low. Many people regard ketosis as a potentially dangerous state, because when ketone levels go very high, as can occur with untreated or poorly controlled type 1 diabetes, a state known as diabetic ketoacidosis, the blood becomes very acidic. Diabetic ketoacidosis can result in dehydration, nausea, vomiting, and in extreme cases, even coma and death. But a ketogenic diet that is properly monitored and controlled has been shown to be helpful in the treatment of epilepsy (a type of seizure disorder) in young children. A ketogenic diet may also be helpful in the treatment of several other disorders, although it is possible that a low-carbohydrate diet, without the production of excess ketones, might be beneficial for some of these disorders as well. Ketogenic diets are usually medically administered and supervised, since these diets can be difficult to follow and may have negative consequences, especially in young children.

Athletes may monitor their total carbohydrate intake for many reasons. Some may be limiting carbohydrate intake to lose weight. Others may be trying to take in extra calories to gain weight, and be following a plan that requires a certain percentage of these calories to come from carbohydrate. Some athletes may be ingesting extra carbohydrate to increase muscle and liver glycogen stores to maximize energy production during sport performance.

19. What is dietary fiber, and why is dietary fiber content listed on the Nutrition Facts panel?

Dietary fiber refers to the components of food that cannot be digested in the stomach or small intestine of human beings. Humans lack the necessary digestive enzymes for breaking down these structures. Once dietary fiber passes into the large intestine, it influences the nature of the material that eventually forms the stools and interacts with the microorganisms that live in the lower portion of the GI tract. Dietary fiber comes primarily from plants, including whole grains, legumes, fruits, and vegetables, and from foods made with these ingredients. Most dietary fibers are types of carbohydrates, which is why dietary fiber content is listed in the carbohydrate section of the Nutrition Facts panel of the food label.

Nutrition scientists refer to the dietary fiber from food as intrinsic or intact fiber. Since these fiber types are a component of the food itself, only the food (not the specific type of fiber) is included on a label's list of ingredients. Dietary fiber also includes processed fiber. Processed fiber refers to ingredients isolated from food or synthetic carbohydrate structures manufactured in the laboratory that, like intact fiber, are not digestible in the upper GI tract. According to the Food and Drug Administration's food labeling regulations, these isolated and synthetic carbohydrates must have been shown to have beneficial health effects (as of 2020). (Before 2020 any of these substances could be included in the fiber content figures on the Nutrition Facts panel.) Consumers may have observed the following isolated or synthetic fibers as ingredients on food labels:

- Beta-glucan soluble fiber
- Psyllium husk
- Cellulose
- Guar gum
- Pectin
- Locust bean gum
- Hydroxypropyl methylcellulose

Newer processed dietary fibers that consumers might see on ingredient lists include:

- Mixed plant cell wall fibers (a broad category that includes fibers like sugar cane fiber and apple fiber, among many others)
- Arabinoxylan
- Alginate
- Inulin and inulin-type fructans
- High amylose starch (resistant starch 2)
- Galactooligosaccharide
- Polydextrose
- Resistant maltodextrin/dextrin

A fiber without a health benefit, such as gum acacia, may be added to a food product. Its grams of carbohydrate would be included in the figure for the food's carbohydrate grams, but not in the figure for the food's dietary fiber grams. (This is a change from the old label, in which all dietary fiber, regardless of whether or not health benefits for that type of fiber had been established, could be included in the dietary fiber figure.)

A food's dietary fiber content is included on the food label because this knowledge helps consumers understand the nature of the food's carbohydrate content (as explained in the previous question on carbohydrates) and because health experts believe most people in the United States should consume diets higher in dietary fiber. Numerous studies have demonstrated that dietary fiber has several beneficial health effects, although these effects vary with the type of fiber consumed. A fiber's behavior in the GI tract is influenced by a number of important variables, including its water solubility (how easily the fiber dissolves in water), viscosity (how much the fiber forms a gel in water), and how much the fiber is fermented (digested) by gut bacteria in the large intestine.

In general, water-soluble fiber attracts water and forms a gel-like mix in the digestive system. This mixture slows stomach emptying, helping eaters feel full longer. Delayed stomach emptying also means that glucose is absorbed from the digestive mass more slowly, thus preventing a rapid rise in blood glucose, which can lead to high blood insulin levels. Water-soluble fiber tends to bind bile acids in the small intestine. Bile is a compound manufactured by the liver and stored in the gall bladder that helps break down dietary fats. Bile acids, an important component of bile, are high in cholesterol. When the bile acids are bound to the fibrous mixture, their cholesterol is not available for reabsorption back into the bloodstream; the bile acids are excreted in the stools. Thus, soluble fiber appears to be beneficial for people trying to reduce blood cholesterol levels.

Water-insoluble fiber provides bulk to the feces and speeds their passage through the GI tract. The rough edges of insoluble fiber, like the fiber found in wheat bran, stimulate the GI tract to propel the food mass along more quickly. Water-insoluble fiber reduces risk of constipation. It should be noted that the functions of water-soluble and water-insoluble fibers as described earlier often overlap; for example, psyllium fiber is primarily water-soluble yet still increases stool bulk.

Fermentable fibers serve as prebiotics, providing food and a healthful environment for the trillions of helpful microorganisms (probiotics) in the GI tract. A diet high in dietary fiber is associated with a healthy intestinal microbiome. Healthful populations of microbiota in the GI tract are associated with better health, including reduced risk of infectious diarrhea, inflammatory bowel conditions, emotional health problems such as depression, and certain types of cancer.

However, fermentable fibers are problematic for some people, because as bacteria break down fermentable fibers, intestinal gas is produced, which can result in bloating and discomfort. Dietary fiber also influences mineral absorption from the GI tract, both increasing and decreasing absorption, depending on the nature of the dietary fiber.

People concerned with consuming dietary fiber for specific health benefits will need more information than can be found on a food label. For example, if a food contains a high amount of dietary fiber, but the fiber is mostly processed digestive-resistant starches, that food may not necessarily be as good as high-fiber foods such as wheat bran for reducing symptoms of constipation.

Currently, adults in the United States consume only about half of the recommended amount of fiber in their diets. The Daily Value for dietary fiber intake is 28 g/day. Fiber intake recommendations are all based on daily calorie intake. All guidelines recommend obtaining 14 g of dietary fiber per 1,000 kcal, regardless of a person's age or sex. The recommended Dietary Reference Intake (DRI) value for fiber is 14 g per 1,000 kcal. For men ages 19–50, 38 g of dietary fiber is recommended per day; the value for men over 50 is 30 g per day, but this difference is only due to a smaller calorie requirement as people age. Similarly, for women ages 19–50, the DRI value is 25 g per day, and for women over 50 it is 21 g per day. Most dietary guidelines encourage people to consume adequate amounts of vegetables, fruits, legumes, and whole grains to promote a healthy intake of dietary fiber, as fiber DRIs were derived from observations of people consuming intact rather than processed fiber.

Like most dietary components, too much fiber, especially in the form of fiber supplements or concentrated sources of fiber such as wheat bran, can be problematic, causing diarrhea and intestinal discomfort. People trying to increase their fiber intake are advised to do so gradually so that their bodies have time to adjust to the new levels.

20. What is meant by the term "total sugars," and why is the amount of total sugars listed on the Nutrition Facts panel?

In common language, many people use the word "sugar" to refer to table sugar, or other types of sugar, like brown sugar or cane sugar. But when chemists use the word "sugar," they are referring to a certain group of carbohydrate chemical structures. (See Question 18.)

Sugars, also known as simple carbohydrates, are relatively small molecules of carbohydrate found naturally in fruits and vegetables, as well as milk. They are especially concentrated in sweeteners such as table sugar (usually made from sugar beets or sugar cane), honey, molasses, and maple syrup. Corn syrup is a sweetener made from the sugar in corn. Many food products contain added sweeteners.

Question 18 explains that the carbohydrate structures in foods are all built from the simplest carbohydrate units called monosaccharides. The term sugars refer to monosaccharides and disaccharides. Monosaccharides contain three to seven carbon atoms. Monosaccharides generally contain carbon, hydrogen, and oxygen in a ratio of two hydrogen atoms and one oxygen atom to each carbon atom, for a molecular formula of $C_nH_{2n}O_n$. The most common monosaccharides in the human diet contain six carbons, and include glucose, fructose, and galactose.

Glucose is the most common monosaccharide found in nature. Glucose provides the types of chemical bonds from which people can capture energy. Glucose is carried in the bloodstream to all cells of the body to be used as an energy production substrate. The term "blood sugar" refers to blood glucose level. Glucose is rarely found as a single unit in foods, but instead forms part of disaccharide structures. Fructose is the sweetest of the monosaccharides and binds with glucose to form the disaccharide sucrose, found in many sweet foods. Galactose is the monosaccharide that is bound to glucose to form lactose, the disaccharide known as milk sugar.

The pentoses are five-carbon monosaccharide molecules. Best known of the pentoses are ribose, a component of RNA and deoxyribose, a component of DNA. The body synthesizes pentoses, so these monosaccharides do not need to be included in the diet.

Monosaccharides also serve as components in genetic material and important coenzymes, such as ATP involved in the metabolic pathways responsible for the production of energy in animals.

The three most common disaccharides in the human diet are sucrose (composed of glucose + fructose), galactose (glucose + lactose), and maltose (two glucose units). Maltose is found in germinating grains, a product of the breakdown of starch.

During digestion, simple sugars, whether a natural part of a food or an added sweetener, are broken down into monosaccharides that are transported into the bloodstream. The liver converts fructose and other monosaccharides into glucose or other molecules, including large chains of glucose called glycogen. Monosaccharides can also be converted into fats.

The amount of total sugars on the Nutrition Facts panel represents all of the sugar structures found in a serving of the labeled food. "Total sugars" on the new label means the same thing as "sugars" on the previous food label. This figure is included on the Nutrition Facts panel because many consumers are concerned about sugar consumption. While most consumers are primarily concerned about "added sugars" (see Question 21), some consumers want to know the total amount of sugar they are consuming. These consumers include people needing to limit all kinds of sugar for health reasons such as diabetes. While a Daily Value is provided for "added sugars," no value is provided for "total sugars."

Some food labels also list another type of sugar, sugar alcohols, on the Nutrition Facts panel. Sugar alcohols, also known as polyols, are a sweetener frequently added to food products. As the name suggests, sugar alcohols have a chemical structure that is very similar to sugar. The alcohol designation refers to specific chemical group (-OH); sugar alcohols do not contain the kind of alcohol found in alcoholic beverages. Examples of sugar alcohol include xylitol, sorbitol, mannitol, erythritol, maltitol, lactitol, isomalt, and hydrogenated starch hydrolysates (HSH). Small amounts of sugar alcohols are found naturally in some fruits and vegetables, but most of the sugar alcohol in food products is produced commercially from sugars and starches. It is added as a sweetener to sugar-free and reduced-sugar products. Sugar alcohols taste sweet but have fewer calories per gram than sugar and do not promote tooth decay. Sugar alcohols are often used in conjunction with non-nutritive sweeteners in food products.

Unlike non-nutritive (artificial) sweeteners (e.g., aspartame), sugar alcohols do supply some calories, about half the calories in the same amount of sugar, depending on the sugar alcohol. Erythritol contains the fewest calories with 0.2 per gram, and HSH contains the most with 3.0 per gram. Sugars have 4 kcal per gram. Sugar alcohols are only partially absorbed into the blood from the small intestine. The portion that is absorbed is converted to glucose slowly, thus triggering little or no insulin response. The portion that is not absorbed passes into the large intestine, where it is fermented by bacteria. Because of the fermentation, overconsumption of sugar alcohols can cause gas, abdominal discomfort, and diarrhea. Products that contain significant amounts of sugar alcohols are required to state "Excess consumption may have a laxative effect" on their packaging.

The Food and Drug Administration (FDA) has ruled that sugar alcohols are not classified as "added sugars." Sugar alcohols must be included on food labels in the ingredient list, but their inclusion on the Nutrition

Facts panel is voluntary. When sugar alcohols are listed separately, they are listed in the "total carbohydrates" section after "added sugars." However, food manufacturers are *required* to list sugar alcohols if a statement is made on the package labeling about the health effects of sugar alcohols or sugars (when sugar alcohols are present in the food). Sugar alcohols are included in the "total carbohydrate" figure.

Foods that contain sugar alcohols but no added sugars can be labeled as "no sugar added" or "sugar-free" foods. Many people mistakenly believe this means they are low calorie and therefore eat them in large quantities. Not only can this lead to gastrointestinal distress, but many of these foods are also highly caloric and contain few beneficial nutrients. People with diabetes must be particularly careful because although normal portions of foods with sugar alcohols do not raise blood sugar levels significantly, levels can rise if large quantities are consumed.

The FDA regulates nutrient content claims related to a product's sugar content. These are defined as follows:

"Sugar-free" and "insignificant source of sugar"—These products contain little sugar.

- Product contains less than 0.5 g of sugar per serving.
- Product contains no added sugar or foods known to contain sugar, unless the ingredient is found on the ingredient list with an asterisk and a statement to the effect "adds a negligible/insignificant amount of sugar."
- Product must also be labeled "a low-calorie food" or "not a low-calorie food," depending on calorie content. This item is to help consumers understand that a low-sugar food may or may not actually be low in calories.

"No sugar added" and "without added sugar"—These products must not have added sugar.

- No type of sugar can be added to the product, and no foods containing sugar can be added to the product.
- The reference food that the product provides an alternative for typically contains sugar.
- Product must also be labeled "not a low-calorie food," unless it meets low-calorie requirements.
- Product must not contain a significant amount of natural sugars.

"Reduced sugar," "less sugar," or "lower in sugar"—These products must contain less sugar than comparable products.

- Product must contain at least 25% less sugar per serving than the reference (standard version of) product.
- Product package must contain a statement next to the reduced sugar claim explaining the difference, such as "contains 25% less sugar than our regular applesauce." Statement must also specify the exact difference in grams of sugar, "sugar content reduced to 12 g per serving compared to 22 g per serving."

21. What is the difference between added sugars and total sugars, and are the health effects different between added sugars and sugars found naturally in food?

A food product's total sugar grams comprise the grams of sugar that occur naturally in the food product ingredients and the grams of sugars that are added during processing. For example, all types of applesauce contain sugars that are found naturally in the apples used as ingredients, but some also have sugar added to make the product sweeter. The grams of "total sugars" would include both types of sugars. The grams of "added sugars" would include only the sugars added.

On a physiological level, the health effects of 1 g of sugar from the sugar bowl appear to be similar to the health effects of 1 g of sugars from a plant food (fruit, vegetable, or grain) or milk. Both types of sugar are absorbed and metabolized by the same biological pathways. However, when people consume sugars as part of a vegetable or fruit, for example, they will obtain many vitamins, minerals, fibers, and other plant compounds (phytochemicals) such as antioxidants, as well as the energy from the sugars. When people consume milk or unsweetened yogurt, they will ingest vitamins, minerals, and protein along with milk's natural sugars. Sugars alone, such as table sugar or brown sugar, have little or no helpful nutrients. Even a supposedly "healthy" sugar such as honey adds little nutritive value to the diet. This is why table sugar and other sweeteners are called "empty calories"; they contain calories but are almost completely empty of nutrients (aside from carbohydrates).

Including "added sugars" on the Nutrition Facts panel was one of the most important changes to the food label. A high intake of sugars is associated with weight gain, obesity, type 2 diabetes, non-alcoholic fatty liver disease, cardiovascular disease, certain types of cancer, and tooth decay. Expert groups, including the Centers for Disease Control and Prevention, the National Academies of Science, the World Health Organization, the Academy of Pediatrics, and the American Heart Association, all agree that people's intake of added sugars should be reduced. Sugar consumption has increased dramatically over the past few decades, and public health professionals hope that more information and education about sugar consumption can help people make better decisions about how much sugar they should consume.

Information about added sugars is given both in grams and in terms of a percent Daily Value (DV). Under the line listing "total sugars," the Nutrition Facts panel will show a line that states "includes X g added sugars," and then give a number for the percent DV. (X indicates the grams of added sugars.) The DV for added sugars is based on the recommendation that no more than 10% of daily kilocalories come from added sugars. Nutrition scientists agree that it is difficult for people to meet their nutrient needs while staying within their calorie limits if they get more than 10% of their calories from added sugars. For people consuming 2,000 kcal/day, this represents 50 g of sugar, the equivalent of about 12.5 teaspoons of table sugar. (Each gram of sugar contributes about 4 kcal.)

The DV for added sugars represents a suggested limit rather than a requirement. No added sugars are necessary in a healthy diet. Except for extremely active people with very high energy needs, most people would benefit from fewer than 50 g of added sugars per day. People consuming fewer than 2,000 kcal/day, people trying to lose weight, and people with type 2 diabetes often decide that 50 g of added sugars per day is too high.

Some people have difficulty controlling their intake of highly processed foods, such as soft drinks, pastries, cookies, and ice cream, which usually contain quite a lot of added sugars. These people may find that sugar consumption decreases feelings of stress and makes them feel better. Indeed, research shows that sugar consumption decreases levels of the stress hormone cortisol and stimulates the reward areas of the brain, the same areas stimulated by addictive drugs. People who have difficulty controlling sugar intake may experience a craving for ultra-processed sugary foods, which can in turn lead to overeating, weight gain, obesity, and obesity-related health problems. Many professionals believe that in such cases, avoidance of added sugars can be helpful.

The Food and Drug Administration (FDA) regulates what ingredients must be included as added sugars. According to the FDA, "These include sugars (free, mono- and disaccharides), sugars from syrups and honey, and sugars from concentrated fruit or vegetable juices that are in excess of what would be expected from the same volume of 100 percent fruit or vegetable juice of the same type. The definition excludes fruit or vegetable juice concentrated from 100 percent fruit juice that is sold to consumers (e.g. frozen 100 percent fruit juice concentrate) as well as some sugars found in fruit and vegetable juices, jellies, jams, preserves, and fruit spreads."

The specific sugars used in food products will be found in the ingredient list on the food label. Over 60 different caloric sweeteners are added to food products. Some product names are recognizable to most consumers: agave, fruit juice, honey, maple syrup, organic cane sugar, molasses, and coconut sugar. Others may be less familiar. Generally, ingredients ending in "-ose," "sugar," or "syrup" are sweeteners: dextrose, high fructose corn syrup, date sugar, and rice syrup, for example.

22. What is protein, and why is protein content listed on the Nutrition Facts panel?

Proteins are nitrogen-containing organic compounds found in all plants and animals. Protein is found throughout the human body, in structures such as muscle and bone; the immune cells that fight infection; the red blood cells that carry oxygen to all parts of the body; neurochemicals and hormones such as serotonin and epinephrine; and the enzymes that regulate biochemical processes such as digestion and energy production. Proteins are composed of smaller units called amino acids. The body uses amino acids to build its own proteins. The body can also break down some amino acids to produce energy, especially during long or heavy bouts of physical activity or when glycogen (a carbohydrate energy molecule found in muscles and the liver) stores are depleted. People obtain protein from food. Protein is plentiful in many foods, especially meat, poultry, seafood, dairy products, nuts, grains, and legumes.

Experts often liken amino acids to letters and proteins to words spelled with those letters. To spell a given word, one must have all of the letters available. The human body needs about 20 different amino acids to make all of the proteins required for life. If humans have an adequate intake of protein in general, they can make 11 of these in sufficient quantities. The other nine must be obtained from the diet on a daily basis. Amino acids that people must obtain from the diet are called essential amino acids. Amino acids that the body can manufacture are called nonessential amino acids. (Of course, these amino acids are still "essential" to life, just not an essential part of the diet.)

Proteins can be quite large, containing thousands of amino acids. These chains of amino acids bend and coil, forming unique three-dimensional structures, depending on the amino acid interactions with one another. The function of a protein molecule often depends on this three-dimensional shape.

All cells need single amino acids to build proteins. Cells are continually breaking down and building proteins. When proteins are broken down, the amino acids are released into the blood stream. Free amino acids are found throughout the body and are collectively referred to as the "amino acid pool." Amino acids from the amino acid pool are used whenever the body needs amino acids for synthesis of proteins.

The body is skilled at reusing amino acids. This recycling of amino acids is called "protein turnover." Protein turnover helps the body meet its amino acids needs. The body synthesizes about 300 g of protein each day; about 200 g of this protein comes from protein turnover. When dietary protein intake is too low to meet the body's needs for amino acids, protein breakdown increases to supply the amino acid pool. This can result in the breakdown of essential body tissues, such as muscles.

The human body can store only a limited amount of amino acids, which is why one must consume foods containing proteins every day. Foods that contain all nine essential amino acids are called complete proteins. These foods include eggs, dairy products, animal flesh (chicken, fish, beef, etc.), animal organs (liver, kidneys, etc.), soybeans, and a few other plant foods. Animal foods more closely match the amino acid profile needed by humans, which is logical since humans are animals, so their composition is similar. However, it is not hard to consume adequate amino acids if one eats a variety of plant sources, as the amino acids that are generally low in grains, for example, are more plentiful in legumes (peas and beans), and vice versa. Combining incomplete proteins (proteins lacking one or more essential amino acids) usually results in an adequate intake of protein. The U.S. Department of Agriculture recommends 0.8 g of protein per kilogram of body weight (or 0.36 g/lb). People who are significantly overweight (in the form of excess body fat) should base their protein intake calculations on a weight that would be healthier for them. This translates to about 54 g per day for a 150 lb (68 kg) person.

Protein content is included on the Nutrient Facts panel because protein is an important nutrient. While experts believe that people in North America generally have adequate intakes of protein, there are some important exceptions. In addition, consumers desire information about their protein intake because many diets emphasize certain macronutrient (protein, carbohydrate, and fat) ratios. People with certain health conditions, such as chronic kidney disease, must limit protein intake and must therefore keep a careful track of their daily protein intake.

What conditions require extra dietary protein?

Several conditions call for extra protein in the diet. Whenever more tissue is being built, more protein is required. Pregnancy, bodybuilding, strength training, and adolescent growth spurts place high demands for amino acids on the body. Lactating mothers are producing a quart or more of milk per day and thus need a higher-than-normal protein intake. People, especially athletes, restricting calories force the body to consume protein for fuel, depleting valuable amino acid stores, and must consume more protein to make up for the loss of other food groups in the diet. (These athletes should also add some carbohydrate to their diet.) Endurance athletes usually burn a certain amount of protein for fuel and need higher protein intakes than sedentary people. Vegetarians, especially vegans (consuming no animal products), will require somewhat higher protein intakes than people who are omnivores (eating all kinds of foods of both plant and animal sources), since much of their protein will be incomplete. Recent studies suggest that older adults may also be healthier with a little extra protein, about 1 g/kg body weight, as these people are at risk for breaking down muscle as they age, and extra dietary protein seems to slow down this process. Any combination of the above (e.g., pregnant vegans) will need more dietary protein, up to 1.2–2 g/kg body weight.

What is the percent Daily Value (%DV) for protein, and why do most food labels not list %DV for protein?

The %DV for protein is 50 g. Percent DV for protein is not required on food labels, although some food manufacturers voluntarily list the %DV per serving on the Nutrition Facts panel. How much a serving of a given food product contributes to the %DV for protein actually varies with the amino acid composition of the protein. The composition is not always known. Since many food products contain incomplete protein, it would be misleading to state that a product contributes a specific percentage of protein toward the DV. Manufacturers whose package labels make a claim about the health effects or the amount of protein (e.g., "high protein" or "low protein") contained in the food must list the %DV for protein per serving in that food, however.

23. What is vitamin D, and why is vitamin D content required on the Nutrition Facts panel?

Vitamin D is a fat-soluble vitamin that is converted into a chemical that functions as a hormone in the body. Vitamin D is actually a group of approximately 10 related chemicals. The two most commonly found in the diet are vitamin D_2 (ergocalciferol) and vitamin D_3 (cholecalciferol). Vitamin D is often referred to as the "sunshine vitamin" as the body can make vitamin D from a precursor in the skin, when the skin is exposed to ultraviolet B (UVB) radiation from the sun. Vitamin D helps to maintain optimal levels of calcium and phosphorus in the blood and helps the body absorb calcium and phosphorus in the small intestine. It encourages normal bone development in children and helps prevent loss of bone mineral and osteoporosis in adults. Adequate levels of vitamin D are associated with better muscle function and reduced risk of falls in older adults compared to adults who are deficient in vitamin D. Adequate vitamin D levels may reduce the risk of some cancers, autoimmune disorders, and heart disease.

People who manufacture adequate amounts of vitamin D with UVB radiation exposure from the sun do not require dietary sources of vitamin D. Vitamin D content is required to be listed on food labels, however, because vitamin D is such an important vitamin and because vitamin D deficiency is fairly common. The 2015–2020 U.S. Dietary Guidelines concluded that vitamin D is a "nutrient of concern" and should therefore be included in the Nutrition Facts panel. Populations in northern latitudes, people with darker skin, older adults, and people who rarely get outdoors often have suboptimal vitamin D levels. People whose skin is always covered by clothing or sunscreens are also at higher risk of vitamin D deficiency. It is important to note that dermatologists caution that sun exposure can increase risk for skin cancer, especially in people with fair skin or genetic predispositions; dermatologists encourage these people to obtain vitamin D from foods rather than from sun exposure.

The Dietary Reference Intake (DRI) for vitamin D is 15 mcg (600 International Units [IU]) per day for people 1–70 years old, and 20 mcg (800 IU) per day for those over 70 years of age. The DRI for pregnant and lactating women is 15 mcg (600 IU). When the Food and Drug Administration (FDA) updated the Daily Values (DV) used on food labels in 2016, the DV for vitamin D for most adults and children over four years old was doubled, from 10 mcg (400 IU) to 20 mcg (800 IU). In addition, the FDA mandated that vitamin D be listed in micrograms (mcg) rather than the previously used IU. However, some manufacturers are choosing to include both units on their labels (1 mcg = 40 IU of vitamin D.)

Vitamin D is rarely found naturally in food. The largest natural supply of vitamin D is fish. Vitamin D can be found in oily fish and cod liver oil. (Cod liver oil is not considered a safe daily supplement because its high levels of vitamin A can cause toxicity.) Egg yolk, butter, and liver also have some vitamin D, although amounts in these foods vary with the diet of the source animal. Some mushrooms contain the plant form of vitamin D. Because there are few food sources of vitamin D, and because many people are unable to make enough vitamin given limitations such as low winter sun exposure, several food sources have been fortified with vitamin D. Milk is fortified with vitamin D in several countries, including the United States and Canada. Most milk in the United States is fortified with 400 IU of vitamin D per quart. Milk was chosen as the vehicle for fortification since vitamin D enhances calcium absorption, and milk contains this mineral. However, most products made with milk (cheese, ice cream, etc.) have not been fortified with vitamin D. Breakfast cereal is also commonly fortified with vitamin D. Vitamin D is added to some brands of soy beverages, orange juice, yogurt, and margarine. Because not all of these food products have added vitamin D, it is important to read food labels. Vitamin D_3 is believed to be more effective as a supplement than vitamin D_2.

Because vitamin D status is influenced by both diet and UVB exposure, studies on dietary intake alone may fail to capture the relationship between vitamin D and health. Measures of serum vitamin D have been assessed in some studies, but sometimes these have been inaccurate. Research on vitamin D and health continues to refine both dietary and serum measures, and to explore the physiological activity of vitamin D.

Many cells in the body have receptors for vitamin D, suggesting that the hormone has a number of regulatory functions and health effects. Vitamin D is best known for its role in helping the body absorb calcium. Calcium is a nutrient that is essential in the formation and proper growth of the bones in the skeletal system. Without adequate amounts of vitamin D osteoporosis can result in adults and rickets can occur in children. Vitamin D works with other hormones to regulate blood calcium level by influencing movement of calcium from the gastrointestinal tract into the bloodstream. If blood calcium levels fall too low and dietary calcium is not adequate, vitamin D also helps to mobilize calcium from bone tissue. This is why vitamin D alone is not sufficient to ensure healthy bones; dietary calcium is required as well.

Emerging evidence suggests that vitamin D also has an impact on skeletal muscle strength and function. Research has found that optimal vitamin D levels are associated with stronger muscles and decreased risk of falling in older adults when compared to adults deficient in vitamin D. Vitamin D may help keep the heart muscle healthy.

Vitamin D receptors are found in the cell membranes of immune cells. Vitamin D is believed to help modulate the activity of a family of immune cells known as T cells. Optimal vitamin D levels are associated with a reduced risk of developing autoimmune diseases such as insulin-dependent diabetes mellitus (type 1 diabetes), multiple sclerosis, and rheumatoid arthritis. Vitamin D may help reduce the frequency of winter upper respiratory tract infections, perhaps by improving immune function.

Vitamin D appears to influence the activity of dividing cells, encouraging cells to differentiate and inhibiting cell proliferation. These influences might help to reduce the risk of cancer, a process in which cells proliferate too rapidly and fail to behave normally. Research suggests that higher intakes of vitamin D and optimal serum vitamin D levels are associated with reduced risk of several types of cancers, although research in this area is still preliminary.

Vitamin D influences insulin metabolism and blood pressure. Adequate vitamin D levels may be helpful for preventing the cardiometabolic syndrome and type 2 diabetes, although other factors play important roles in these disorders as well.

Experts are at present unclear as to what levels of serum vitamin D are optimal for good health, although recommendations generally range from 20 to 30 ng/ml. Some health providers recommend vitamin D supplementation based on blood tests, while others simply recommend that individuals consume the DRI daily. Understanding the effect of vitamin D on various health outcomes is complicated because it works in conjunction with other nutrients, such as calcium, magnesium, vitamin A, and vitamin K. Individuals working to maintain optimal vitamin D status should be sure to achieve an adequate dietary intake of these other nutrients as well.

Sun exposure does not cause vitamin D toxicity, but toxicity can result from a higher-than-recommended intake of dietary supplements. Too much vitamin D in the body can lead to an abnormally high level of calcium in the blood, which over time can lead to calcium deposits in soft tissues such as the heart, lungs, blood vessels, and kidneys. While vitamin D toxicity is unlikely at intakes up to 10,000 IU per day, because of the severity of toxicity effects, the tolerable upper intake level has been set fairly low, at 4,000 IU per day.

24. What is calcium, and why is calcium content required on the Nutrition Facts panel?

Calcium is the most abundant mineral found in the human body and plays a key role in a variety of functions. Calcium is stored in bones and teeth, and 99% of the body's calcium can be found in these structures.

In bones, calcium becomes part of a crystalline structure called hydroxy-apatite. This structure surrounds formations that comprise collagen and other proteins. Cells known as osteoblasts and osteoclasts work to form and dismantle bone, respectively. Calcium can be released from bone into the bloodstream when it is needed in other body tissues and to maintain a constant blood calcium concentration. The process of releasing calcium from bone is regulated by vitamin D, parathyroid hormone, and the hormone calcitonin. Calcium performs many other functions as well. In neurons, action potentials travel down axons, which triggers a calcium release. This calcium release causes vesicles within the neuron to release neurotransmitter into the synapse, to propagate the nerve signal throughout the body. In muscles, the neurotransmitter acetylcholine is released onto the muscle cells, which leads to downstream calcium release within the muscle fibers. The calcium molecules bind to proteins that are part of the contractile machinery, controlling muscle contraction. Calcium can also bind to the protein calmodulin. The calcium-calmodulin complex plays a part in regulating secretion, cell division, and the movement of cilia. Calcium is important for blood clotting.

Calcium is found in many foods but is most plentiful in dairy products such as milk, yogurt, and cheese. It is also found in many vegetables, including Chinese cabbage, kale, and broccoli as well as in fish with edible bones. Grains, such as bread, pasta, and cereals, naturally have very little calcium in single servings, but since they are often eaten in large quantities they can be a helpful source of calcium for some people. Grains, milk substitutes such as soy "milk," and other foods are commonly fortified with calcium and therefore can become good dietary sources of the mineral. Many people take in calcium citrate or calcium carbonate in the form of dietary supplements.

Calcium is required on the Nutrition Facts panel because the 2015–2020 U.S. Dietary Guidelines flagged calcium as a "nutrient of concern," because the nutrient has many important associations with health and people often fall sort of reaching healthful intake levels. In addition, many consumers are concerned about their calcium intakes. They use the calcium information on food labels to make decisions about which products to purchase and to keep an eye on their calcium intake levels. While calcium is important for many functions, its role in bone density is what most commonly prompts people to try to meet their calcium requirements in order to maintain good bone strength and integrity, and to possibly prevent or at least delay the onset of bone mineral loss as they age, a condition that can lead to a bone disease called osteoporosis. On the other hand, some people have been advised to limit calcium intake to prevent painful calcium deposits in the kidney, a condition known as kidney stones. Food labels can help them avoid consuming too much calcium.

The current Daily Value (DV) for calcium is 1,300 mg/day, which is 300 mg/day higher than the previous DV of 1,000 mg/day. The Daily Recommended Intake (DRI) for calcium varies with sex, age, and stage of life. Throughout life bones are continuously being remodeled, but during times of growth more bone is being built than broken down, so calcium intake needs to be increased. The DRI for calcium suggests that both males and females 9–18 years old consume 1,300 mg/day, since bone is being formed. The DV reflects the needs of this important age group. During early and middle adulthood bones reach a peak bone mass (ca. 30 years old) and at this time the rates of building and breakdown are the same. For people 19–50 years old, the DRI is 1,000 mg/day of calcium. The DRI for pregnant and lactating women is 1,300 mg/day. Calcium is an essential ingredient in breast milk, and it is hoped that adequate dietary calcium will prevent calcium loss from the bones in mothers who are breastfeeding.

In aging adults and postmenopausal women, more bone is being broken down than being built. Absorption of calcium may also decline with age, so calcium recommendations for these groups are a little higher than those of younger adults. Women over 50 and men over 70 are recommended to consume 1,200 mg of calcium per day.

Some groups are more prone to low calcium intake or absorption. Young women with amenorrhea (lack of menstrual cycle), either due to low caloric intake or too much exercise, have lower calcium absorption (because of lower estrogen levels), which puts them at risk for low bone density. Lactose intolerance and vegan diets (which prohibit the consumption of dairy products) may be associated with a low calcium intake. Not only can calcium deficiency be caused by malabsorption or low intake, but it can also be due to increased excretion from the body. Calcium excretion in the urine is increased with high protein and high sodium intakes. Excretion can also be affected by some medicines.

Too much or too little calcium can influence a wide range of health issues. One of the most common health problems associated with calcium is low bone density. Adequate levels of calcium must be consumed to reach peak bone density by age 30. If not enough calcium is absorbed to replace bone calcium loss, low bone mineral levels and, eventually, osteoporosis may develop. It is important to note, however, that bone metabolism is complex, and dietary calcium availability is only one of many factors that influence the development of osteoporosis. Osteoporosis, which means "porous bones," is a bone disease characterized by gradually declining bone mass. As the mineral and protein content of bones is lost, the bones become less dense, with larger open spaces in them. As the bones become more porous, they also become more fragile. This weakening of the bones can lead to fractures, most commonly in the spine, hip, and wrist. Fractures are debilitating injuries, especially in older adults. About half of all women and a fourth of all men over age 50 experience a fracture at some time. Generally, women who are 50 years of age or older (postmenopausal) and men over the age of 70 years are most susceptible to significant decreases in bone mineral content, also known as bone mineral density (BMD). Osteoporosis is a silent disease and often remains undetected until a person suffers a fracture or notices a loss of height because of bone loss in the spinal column.

Peak bone mass is achieved in young adulthood and begins to decline around the age of 40, at which time both men and women lose bone mass at a rate of about 0.5% per year. In the five years following menopause, women lose bone mass at a faster rate, even with a good diet and plenty of physical activity. After these five years, bone loss returns to a slower pace.

A variety of risk factors are associated with osteoporosis. Women are more likely than men to develop osteoporosis. White and Asian women are at greater risk than other groups. People who are underweight are also generally more at risk than those at normal weight, especially at an older age. A family history of osteoporosis is a strong risk factor. The sex hormones estrogen and testosterone protect against osteoporosis, so low levels of these, as it occurs with aging, menopause, or disruption of the menstrual cycle in women, increase the rate of bone mineral loss. Poor digestive function can reduce the absorption of nutrients such as calcium that are important for bone health. A poor diet can also increase risk for osteoporosis. Physical activity that applies force to the bones, such as walking and strength training, increases bone density. Because peak bone mass is attained in young adulthood, osteoporosis prevention ideally begins in childhood and adolescence with a healthful diet and adequate vigorous physical activity.

Osteoporosis is diagnosed when BMD reaches a critically low level. While many medications are available to help slow down bone loss, all have side effects and result in only minor gains in BMD. Several lifestyle factors, including regular physical activity and good nutrition, can help slow down the rate of bone loss in midlife, and possibly in old age as well.

Therefore, it makes sense for all people, especially those at risk for osteo-porosis, to be physically activity and consume a healthful diet, including adequate calcium intake.

Nutrition can impact rates of bone mineral deposition and loss throughout the lifespan. Although genetics, age, and hormonal status are much stronger risk factors than diet, a variety of dietary issues including calcium and vitamin D intake, protein intake, and the intake of other nutrients and dietary components affect bone metabolism. Consumption of cola beverages and a high consumption of soft drinks in general have been linked to lower BMD. Researchers speculate that people who drink several soft drinks per day may drink less milk or other more healthful beverages. Cola beverages appear to be most harmful, perhaps because they contain phosphoric acid. Ingesting too much phosphorus and too little calcium interferes with calcium absorption, as phosphorus binds to calcium, making it unavailable.

Studies show that getting adequate calcium may have other health effects as well, including reducing risk of hypertension. A diet with ade-quate calcium, potassium, and magnesium appears to help buffer some-what the negative effect of sodium on resting blood pressure.

Some studies have suggested that meeting the Daily Value for calcium consumption lowers the risk of colon and rectal cancers as well as reduces the risk of nonmalignant colon tumors. Calcium binds to bile acids (secreted by the liver to aid the digestion of fat) and other fats in the gas-trointestinal (GI) tract, which may reduce the ability of the fats to dam-age cells in the lining of the colon. However, because some studies suggest that a high calcium intake increases the risk of prostate cancer, the Amer-ican Cancer Society does not recommend that people consume more than the Daily Value of calcium for the purpose of cancer prevention.

Many studies have attempted to elucidate the effect of calcium on cardiovascular disease (CVD). It is thought that by decreasing the intes-tinal absorption of lipids, relatively high levels of calcium may decrease the risk of CVD. However, several recent studies found that men who ingested greater than 1,000 mg/day of supplemental calcium had a 20% increase in their risk of CVD. Results for calcium intake in women have been mixed. Researchers agree that at some level, high intakes of cal-cium from medications and supplements can lead to hypercalcemia, high blood calcium levels. Hypercalcemia can lead to increased blood clotting, calcification of the blood vessels, and stiffening of the arteries, all of which contribute to cardiovascular disease. Experts recommend that calcium be obtained from food rather than supplements when pos-sible. In addition, upper limits for calcium have been set at fairly low levels to discourage high consumption of calcium. U.S. and Canadian recommendations for upper limits of calcium intake are 2,000 mg/day for people over 51, 2,500 mg/day for people 19–50, and 3,000 mg/day for people 9–18.

Calcium may interact with the certain medications. It can reduce the absorption of bisphosphates, fluoroquinolones and tetracycline antibiotics, and levothyroxine. Diuretics have also been found to decrease calcium excretion in the kidneys, which increases blood calcium concentration. Glucocorticoids, mineral oil, laxatives, and antacids with magnesium or aluminum can lead to reduced blood calcium levels.

The amount of calcium that is absorbed from foods and supplements depends on the calcium source, amount taken at one time, age, vitamin D availability, and other food components. On average, people absorb about 30% of the calcium they consume. The DRIs and Daily Values take this into account, so the recommended intake values reflect the knowledge that people's absorption of calcium (and many other nutrients) is limited. Increased levels of vitamin D allow for more calcium to be absorbed from the GI tract. Absorption rate is highest during peak growth times of life, including infancy, puberty, and pregnancy. As people age, their ability to absorb calcium declines.

25. What is iron, and why is iron content required on the Nutrition Facts panel?

Iron is an essential mineral that performs many important functions in the human body. Iron enables the body to produce the important oxygen-carrying compounds hemoglobin and myoglobin. Hemoglobin is a protein in red blood cells that transports oxygen, and myoglobin is a protein that serves a similar function in muscles. Oxygen is required for the production of energy from food. Many enzymes in the body require iron to function properly, and iron is essential for immune system and brain function.

Iron content is important on the Nutrition Facts panel because iron deficiency is a common problem. More recently, iron overload, or consuming and storing too much iron, has been recognized as a serious problem as well. Therefore, many people are concerned about their iron intake and use the information on iron content provided by food labels.

Iron deficiency is the most common nutrient deficiency worldwide, and in North America. Groups most affected include young children, women of childbearing age, pregnant women, and older adults. Vegetarians are also at risk for iron deficiency. Rates of iron deficiency in the United

States and Canada are highest in older adults (up to 20%), but these rates are often due to concurrent illness as well as low iron intake.

Iron deficiency can have serious outcomes, especially in young children and pregnant women. In young children, iron deficiency can cause delays in both motor and cognitive development, as well as behavioral problems. In pregnant women, iron deficiency increases risk of preterm delivery and low birth weight babies. (Low birth weight babies are more likely to have health problems than those born at a healthy weight.) Iron deficiency often results from inadequate dietary iron, but it can also be caused by several other factors, including problems with iron absorption, increased iron loss, and increased iron requirements.

In children and young adults, iron deficiency most commonly results from inadequate levels of iron in the diet. Dietary iron exists in two forms: heme and nonheme iron. Nonheme iron is found in plant sources, dairy products, eggs, iron supplements, and iron-fortified food. Heme iron is located within hemoglobin, and therefore it is found only in meat sources; however, meats also contain nonheme iron. Meats such as chicken, beef, and fish, for example, contain approximately 60% of their iron as nonheme iron. Heme iron is more readily absorbed in the body, but a majority of the iron supplied by the typical diet is nonheme. In general, people in good health absorb about 25–35% of the heme iron and about 2–20% of the nonheme iron in their diet. A lack of heme iron sources in the diet greatly reduces overall iron intake and absorption, as nonheme iron is best absorbed when consumed in a mixed diet that includes both animal and plant foods. The values for iron on the Nutrition Facts panel include both types of iron and do not indicate whether the iron contained in the food product is heme or nonheme. However, consumers can assume only products containing meat would contain heme iron.

The amount of iron absorbed from the diet depends on many factors in addition to iron intake. Some foods such as tea, coffee, whole grains, legumes, and milk or dairy products contain substances that decrease the amount of nonheme iron absorbed. Calcium supplements also can decrease the amount of iron absorbed at a meal. Gastrointestinal disorders can affect the body's ability to absorb iron (and other nutrients) from food. Celiac disease, for example, reduces the ability of the small intestine to absorb nutrients. Pathogens such as hookworm and schistosomiasis, which commonly are found in many middle- and low-income countries, increase a person's risk of iron deficiency by decreasing iron absorption. Fortunately, increased iron need often increases iron absorption. Increased iron absorption also occurs during periods of growth, and during menstruation and pregnancy. Foods and supplements high in vitamin C increase iron absorption.

Iron requirements are highest for pregnant women (27 mg/day), since iron is required for the increased blood volume that develops during pregnancy. Menstrual blood loss leads to higher iron needs in women who menstruate regularly, typically women 13–50 years old. People experiencing blood loss from a health problem such as a bleeding ulcer may also become iron deficient.

Iron deficiency can be diagnosed by measuring the body's iron stores, most commonly, testing hemoglobin and hematocrit via a blood test. Hematocrit is the ratio of the volume of red blood cells to the total blood volume. Without enough available iron, the body does not produce adequate amount of hemoglobin and, thus, not enough red blood cells. Low values on these tests result in a diagnosis of iron-deficiency anemia, the most common form of anemia.

Iron overload generally results from genetic disorders that cause excess iron absorption. Sometimes iron overload occurs because of a very high intake of iron over a long period of time, usually from supplements rather than from foods. The most common cause of iron overload is a genetic disorder called hemochromatosis. This disorder is most common in Caucasian people of Northern European descent, where it affects about 4 in 1,000 people, and is rare in other groups. This disorder develops when the gene for hemochromatosis is inherited from both parents. With this disorder, there is a gradual buildup of iron in the organs, including the heart, liver, and pancreas. Interestingly, some people with this disorder do not experience problems, while others show severe symptoms such as cirrhosis, heart problems, or diabetes, usually after age 40. People with this disorder should check iron values on food labels to get an idea of how much iron they are consuming. Since the only way the body can reduce iron levels is through blood loss, people with iron overload disorders are advised to donate blood regularly. Men and nonmenstruating women are advised to only take iron supplements when advised to do so because they have been diagnosed with iron deficiency by their health care providers.

It is important to note that the Daily Value (DV) used for calculating percent DV for iron on the Nutrition Facts panel represents the iron RDA for females ages 19–50, which is 18 mg/day. The RDA for men and older women is only 8 mg/day. This means that a serving of a food product that, according to the Nutrition Facts panel, supplies 20% of the DV for iron supplies about 3.6 mg of iron. In fact, 3.6 mg of iron would supply about 45% of the RDA for an adult male or for a female over 50.

26. What is potassium, and why is potassium content required on the Nutrition Facts panel?

Potassium is an electrolyte critical to many cellular and electrical functions in the human body. In general, potassium plays important roles in helping to regulate the body's acid-base balance, build muscles, synthesize proteins, manage fluid balance, metabolize carbohydrates, and regulate electrical activity of the heart and nerves. Potassium is found in a wide variety of food sources. Fruits with significant amounts of potassium include bananas, kiwis, prunes, dried apricots, and citrus fruits. Vegetables such as potatoes with their skins, broccoli, peas, lima beans, and squashes all contain potassium. All meats have potassium, as do several fish sources, including salmon, cod, flounder, and sardines. Potassium is also found in yogurt, milk, nuts, and soy products.

Potassium content is required on food labels because the 2015–2020 U.S. Dietary Guidelines listed potassium as a "nutrient of concern." The Daily Value (DV) used on food labels is an older Dietary Reference Intake (DRI) level of potassium for adults: 4,700 mg/day. (DRIs for potassium were lowered in 2019, as the Food and Nutrition Board changed the value to reflect levels designed to prevent deficiency symptoms rather than levels that might possibly prevent hypertension and other chronic health problems.) Dietitians advocate that individuals increase potassium intake by consuming dietary sources of potassium rather than taking supplements, unless prescribed by a doctor.

A relatively high potassium dietary intake level has been found to provide cardioprotective effects. Dietary potassium helps to temper the negative effect of dietary sodium on blood pressure. High blood pressure, also known as hypertension, is a major risk factor for heart disease and stroke, leading causes of death in the United States and many other countries. Many studies have found a relationship between dietary potassium intake and significant reductions in resting blood pressure. In populations that consume high amounts of fruits and vegetables the rate of hypertension is as low as 1% compared to industrialized countries with high intakes of processed foods and hypertension rates of 33%. Researchers have suggested if consumers in industrialized countries increased their potassium levels, rates of hypertension would decrease significantly. Because of the strength of this research, the Food and Drug Administration (FDA) has approved the following health claim for food labels: "Diets containing foods that are a good source of potassium and that are low in sodium may reduce the risk of high blood pressure and stroke."

Potassium's alkalinity may help combat age-related muscle mass loss. Several studies have found that higher levels of potassium consumption are associated with a greater percentage of lean body mass in healthy older men and women. The acidosis that occurs gradually with age and contributes to several health problems in later adulthood could be neutralized by potassium-rich alkaline foods, like fruits and vegetables. Potassium's alkalinity could also help maintain bone mineral density (BMD). Research that has compared subjects' dietary intakes of potassium to BMD measures has revealed positive associations between potassium intake and BMD measures. High levels of acidity can result in excessive calcium excretion leading to more fragile and less healthy bones.

Reducing calcium excretion through increased potassium intake may also reduce risk of kidney stones. Dietary potassium levels appear to be inversely related to kidney stone development over time. It has been suggested that potassium's ability to reduce calcium excretion might be responsible for this association.

A low blood level of potassium is called hypokalemia. Typically, hypokalemia results from excessive potassium loss in urine and not from low levels in the diet. The most common causes include use of diuretics, kidney diseases, and prolonged vomiting or diarrhea. The symptoms of hypokalemia are weakness, constipation, fatigue, muscle cramps, and arrhythmias.

There is no set upper limit (UL) for potassium. Hyperkalemia, high blood potassium level, can be a life-threatening condition. However, hyperkalemia is almost always caused by kidney disease rather than diet, so treatment targets managing the underlying medical condition. Doctors recommend individuals with some types of kidney problems to not consume excessive amounts of potassium-rich foods, so being able to access potassium levels on food labels is especially important for these people. Hyperkalemia can also be caused pharmacologically by medications such as ACE-inhibitors and blood thinners. Symptoms of hyperkalemia include weakness, muscle fatigue, nausea, and arrhythmias.

It is especially important for people to achieve a healthful potassium intake by eating food, rather than trying to reach their DRI with supplements. Most dietary supplement manufacturers limit the amount of potassium in their products to less than 100 mg for two reasons. First, the FDA has stated that some oral drug products, including potassium chloride enteric-coated tablets, containing more than 99 mg of potassium are not safe, as their use is associated with small bowel lesions. Second, the FDA mandates that some potassium salts (typically marketed as salt substitutes for sodium-containing salt) containing more than 99 mg per tablet be labeled with a warning about the product link to small bowel lesions. (The FDA does not currently require a warning on dietary supplements containing more than 99 mg of potassium, and lesions do not appear to be associated with dietary supplements of potassium, but manufacturers are concerned that such a situation could develop.)

Unlike some minerals, potassium is absorbed efficiently from the diet; people appear to absorb about 95% of the potassium they consume.

27. What is vitamin A, and why is vitamin A no longer required on the Nutrition Facts panel?

Vitamin A is a fat-soluble vitamin that facilitates many critical physiological processes in the body. Like all vitamins, vitamin A is an organic compound that is necessary in small amounts for normal growth, development, and maintenance of basic functions. Unlike water-soluble vitamins, which are excreted from the body when not used, fat-soluble vitamins are stored in the liver and fatty tissues. Vitamin A comes in two different forms: preformed vitamin A and provitamin A. Preformed vitamin A is found in animal products in the form of retinoids. Retinoids are a group of chemical compounds that include retinol, retinal, and retinoic acid. Provitamin A is found in plant products in the form of carotenoids, which are a group of over 600 plant pigments found in red, orange, and deep-yellow fruits and vegetables, as well as many dark, leafy greens. Several forms of carotenoids can be converted into vitamin A in the human body, including beta-carotene, alpha-carotene, and beta-cryptoxanthin. Other carotenoids, including xanthophyll, zeaxanthin, and lycopene, may be beneficial to health but are not converted into vitamin A. Once ingested, both preformed vitamin A and provitamin A are metabolized into retinal and retinoic acid, which are the active forms of vitamin A. They are stored in the form of retinyl esters, mainly in the liver.

Vitamin A plays many important roles in the body, some of which are well understood, and others less so. The most clearly understood is vitamin A's role in vision. In fact, the term "retinoids" comes from their importance to the retina. Vitamin A helps the eye see images, distinguish colors, and adjust to dim light. When light enters the eye, it enters through the cornea, travels to the lens, and then hits the retina. The light combines with retinal located in the retina, and this reaction sends a signal to the brain that is interpreted as an image. Without vitamin A, vision deteriorates. Night blindness, or the inability to see in dim light, is a common symptom of vitamin A deficiency. If vitamin A deficiency continues, the cells along the cornea lose their ability to produce tears and mucus, which causes the eye to become dry. Dry eyes can be scratched by dirt and other particles, leading to infection. This condition is called xerophthalmia, and the eye may develop a clouding of the cornea, ultimately causing blindness.

Vitamin A also plays an important role in the reproduction and growth of cells. Cell differentiation, the process through which immature cells develop into specialized cells, requires vitamin A. It is particularly important for epithelial cells, which line the lungs, digestive tract, eyes, and skin, and for immune cells called *T lymphocytes*. Vitamin A deficiency, therefore, decreases the body's immune response. Vitamin A also plays a role in breaking down and building bone tissue, reproduction, and in skin health.

Achieving an adequate intake of vitamin A is not often a problem for North American adults who maintain a balanced diet, although vitamin A deficiencies are seen in elderly and chronically ill individuals. Vitamin A deficiency (VAD) is most commonly found in underdeveloped countries where poor nutrition is a major health concern; children and pregnant and lactating women are particularly at risk. The symptoms of VAD include night blindness, xerophthalmia, dry skin and hair, and decreased ability to fight infection. Treatment for less serious cases of VAD involves a diet full of foods rich in vitamin A, whereas more serious cases require high levels of vitamin A supplementation.

Dietary recommendations for vitamin A are sometimes a source of confusion for consumers. The Daily Value (DV) for vitamin A used on food labels is given in older units, called International Units, or IU, and is 5,000 IU. The recommended dietary intake of vitamin A given on Dietary Reference Intake tables of the Food and Nutrition Board is expressed in micrograms (mcg), 900 mcg per day for adult males and 700 mcg per day for adult females. Microgram values represent the vitamin A activity of retinol. Since foods with carotenoids vary in their vitamin A potential, depending on the types and amounts of the carotenoids they contain, expression of vitamin A activity is given in nutrition sources as retinol activity equivalents (RAE); 1 RAE = 1 mcg of retinol. There is no simple conversion factor for changing IU to mcg, as the conversion factors vary with the type of vitamin A, as follows:

1 IU retinol = 0.3 mcg RAE
1 IU beta-carotene from dietary supplements = 0.15 mcg RAE
1 IU beta-carotene from food = 0.05 mcg RAE
1 IU alpha-carotene or beta-cryptoxanthin = 0.025 mcg RAE

The majority of vitamin A is absorbed in the intestine and travels with fats into cells; therefore, it is absorbed best when eaten with fat. Vitamin A is stored in the liver and fatty tissue until specific carriers transport it where it is needed throughout the body.

The best sources of preformed vitamin A are animal liver and fish oils, while the best sources of pro-vitamin A are leafy greens, orange and yellow fruits and vegetables, and tomato products. Whole milk is another good source of vitamin A. The process of creating lower fat milk removes much of the vitamin A; however, low fat and skim milk are often fortified with vitamin A. Unlike water-soluble vitamins, fat-soluble vitamins are not lost through cooking. In fact, chopping carotenoid-containing foods and cooking them in oil generally increases their bioavailability.

Because vitamin A is important for cell growth and differentiation, research has focused on its potential role in cancer reduction or prevention. However, studies have had mixed results. In some cases, beta-carotene and retinyl palmitate supplements appear to correlate with lower levels of cancer, but other studies have not replicated these findings. Vitamin A can also reduce mortality due to measles and pneumonia in children as well as help prevent macular degeneration in aging populations.

Excess intake of vitamin A, called hypervitaminosis A, may result in a myriad of negative effects, including blurred vision, headache, irritability, nausea, loss of appetite, hair and skin changes, and mild fever. Excess alcohol consumption in conjunction with excess vitamin A supplementation may result in liver damage. The tolerable upper intake levels (UL) of vitamin A in adult males and females is 3,000 mcg per day. Hypervitaminosis A can be caused by excess short-term or long-term consumption of vitamin A, generally in supplement form. Because the body converts beta-carotene into vitamin A only as needed, beta-carotene is a safe source of vitamin A. Symptoms of hypervitaminosis A can usually be reversed without lasting effects by stopping the excess intake of vitamin A.

Vitamin A is no longer required on the Nutrition Facts panel because nutrient deficiencies for the vitamin are relatively rare in the United

States, and the need to urge consumers to increase their intake of this vitamin is not as strong as that for the nutrients that have replaced vitamins A and C on the label. In the decades leading up to the early 1990s, when the previous food label was developed, nutrition scientists had an interest in the idea that a high intake of and possibly supplementation with vitamin A and the carotenoids might help to prevent cancer. The experts designing the Nutrition Facts panel wanted to prompt consumers to look for foods rich in vitamin A, and thus vitamin A was included on the Nutrition Facts panel. However, over the years evidence supporting the association of vitamin A intake and cancer prevention has not been compelling. Scientists now believe that urging consumers to consume a larger amount and variety of plant foods, especially fruits and vegetables, is a better approach to cancer prevention. Food labels may voluntarily list the vitamin A content of their product, so consumers still see vitamin A listed on some labels.

28. What is vitamin C, and why is vitamin C no longer required on the Nutrition Facts panel?

Vitamin C, also known as ascorbic acid, is a water-soluble vitamin. Like all vitamins, vitamin C is an organic compound that is necessary in small amounts for normal growth, development, and maintenance of basic functions. Vitamin C's functions include assisting in collagen production, intensifying the body's absorption of iron, aiding in wound healing, and maintaining healthy bones and teeth. The body needs vitamin C to help produce many essential compounds such as the neurotransmitter serotonin, bile salts, thyroid hormone, steroid hormones, and parts of the DNA molecule.

Diets rich in vitamin C have been associated with reduced risk of heart disease in some studies, although it is unclear whether vitamin C is the causative agent, or simply a marker for diets rich in fruits and vegetables. Vitamin C is known to help the body's immune system by supporting the function of immune cells. Companies often market their vitamin C supplementation products as prevention and/or treatment methods against the common cold. Several scientific studies have questioned the truth of these claims, however.

Vitamin C also works as an antioxidant. As an antioxidant, vitamin C helps eliminate free radicals from the body. Free radicals are molecules that have a single electron, making the molecules highly reactive as they "look" for another electron to complete the incomplete valence. In cells, free radicals can take electrons from other molecules, including those in important structures such as DNA and cell membranes. By donating electrons to stabilize free radicals, antioxidants in the human body help to prevent or delay some types of cell damage.

Free radicals come from a variety of sources. Individuals can be exposed to free radicals via the environment from sources such as cigarette smoke, air pollution, and sunlight. Free radicals also are produced in the body during normal oxidative metabolism, the process by which energy is produced in the mitochondria from oxygen and the fuel precursors carbohydrates, proteins, and fat. When the human body converts food into energy, unstable molecules are formed as part of the natural process of breaking down food. Scientists believe free radicals can trigger cell damage, and may be partly responsible for the development and/or progression of diseases such as cancer, cardiovascular diseases, diabetes, Alzheimer's disease, Parkinson's disease, cataracts, and age-related macular degeneration.

Antioxidants come from many dietary sources. The vitamins E and C display antioxidant activity. Many phytochemicals behave as antioxidants. Phytochemicals are substances in plants that promote health but are not technically vitamins or minerals. (To qualify as a vitamin or mineral, lack of the substance in the diet must cause deficiency symptoms.) Phytochemicals known for their antioxidant potential include carotenoids such as beta-carotene, lycopene, and lutein. In addition, the human body produces its own antioxidant substances to counteract free radical production.

Vitamin C is found in many fruits and vegetables such as apples, asparagus, berries, broccoli, cabbage, melons, cauliflower, citrus fruits, kiwi, dark leafy greens, peppers, potatoes, and tomatoes. Breads, grains, cereals, and juices are often fortified with vitamin C. Fresh, raw fruits and vegetables supply the highest amounts of vitamin C. Because vitamin C is water-soluble, cooking foods in water decreases the vitamin content. To preserve this vitamin content, best practices suggest decreasing cooking time as much as possible, using minimal amounts of water, and draining the water immediately after cooking.

The Daily Value (DV) for vitamin C, 60 mg, is a little lower than the current Dietary Reference Intakes (DRI) established by the Food and Nutrition Board. DRI for vitamin C for adult men 19 and older is 90 mg and for adult females 19 and older is 75 mg. Because smokers are at a higher risk for vitamin C deficiency, their DRI increases an extra 35 mg. A diet with plenty of fruits and vegetables allows most individuals to achieve their vitamin C DRI. Once daily consumption reaches around 200 mg, through any combination of foods or supplements, vitamin C has reached its maximum absorption capacity and additional intake will result in loss via the urine. Mega dosing, taking too much vitamin C, may cause headaches, diarrhea, nausea, insomnia, bloating, abdominal cramping, heartburn, vomiting, and frequent urination. Some research suggests that individuals at an increased risk for kidney stones should not consume high levels of vitamin C. Excess vitamin C is converted into oxalate, which is a component of a very common type of kidney stone, calcium oxalate.

Vitamin C is no longer required on the Nutrition Facts panel because nutrient deficiencies for the vitamin are relatively rare in the United States, and the need to urge consumers to increase their intake of this vitamin is not as strong as that for the nutrients that have replaced vitamins C and A on the label. In the decades leading up to the early 1990s, when the previous food label was developed, nutrition scientists had an interest in the idea that a high intake of and possibly supplementation with vitamin C and other antioxidants might help to prevent a number of health problems. The experts designing the Nutrition Facts panel wanted to prompt consumers to look for foods rich in vitamin C, and thus vitamin C was included on the Nutrition Facts panel. However, over the years evidence supporting the association of vitamin C intake and the prevention of health problems such as the common cold, heart disease, and cancer has not been compelling. Scientists now believe that urging people to consume a larger amount and variety of plant foods, especially fruits and vegetables, is a better approach to an adequate intake of antioxidants and disease prevention. Food labels may voluntarily list the vitamin C content of their product, so consumers still see vitamin C listed on some labels.

Ingredients and Allergens

29. How can the ingredient list be useful to consumers?

Every food product package must include an ingredient list. The ingredient list is useful for many reasons. It is especially critical for anyone wishing to avoid certain ingredients. People with allergies or food intolerances rely on the ingredient list to avoid triggering an allergic response or digestive discomfort. Such responses range in severity from annoying to life-threatening. While a handful of the most common allergens must be listed in a mandated allergen statement, many other food ingredients can cause allergies or other symptoms in susceptible people as well. Since these are not listed in the allergen statement, the ingredient list must be accurate and complete.

The ingredient list is also important for people trying to avoid certain foods for health reasons. For example, while the value for trans fat on the Nutrition Facts panel may say "0," savvy consumers realize that there may still be a small amount (less than 0.5 g per serving) of trans fat in the product. Finding hydrogenated or partially hydrogenated oils in the ingredient list tells people that indeed a small amount of trans fat is likely present in the product. Sometimes people must avoid certain ingredients while they are taking a medication, or because they are on some sort of special elimination diet to diagnose or treat a health problem, and they rely on ingredient lists to figure out what they may or may not eat.

Some people avoid certain ingredients for religious or philosophical reasons. They rely on the ingredient list to determine whether the food contains animal products, for example, if they follow a vegan diet.

All ingredients in the food product must be listed in order from the highest to the lowest in weight. Knowing this fact can help consumers read between the lines regarding product advertising. For example, a breakfast cereal package might say something like "part of a balanced breakfast," and yet have sugar listed as one of the top ingredients. Checking the Nutrition Facts panel for added sugars can further help people make decisions about how that product fits into a healthy breakfast.

Many consumers are aware that food product manufacturers can manipulate recipes so that less desirable ingredients (from the average consumer's point of view) appear farther down the list. This is commonly seen with added sugars. The recipe for a snack bar, for example, might use several different kinds of sweeteners. This allows the more healthful ingredients, such as grains and nuts, to appear as the first ingredients. Again, checking the added sugars' figure is helpful.

The Food and Drug Administration (FDA) spells out in detail how certain ingredients may or may not be listed. For example, individual spices do not need to be listed; the ingredient list can simply say "spices." Caffeine added to a food product must be listed, but when an ingredient, such as coffee, that naturally contains caffeine is added to a food, such as coffee ice cream, caffeine need not be listed as an ingredient.

Special rules also apply to flavorings, colorings, and chemical preservatives as to how each should be named. Most flavorings need not be individually listed. The ingredient list may simply state "artificial flavor." The same goes for some food colorings, although many food colorings (e.g., "FD&C Yellow No. 5") must be listed by name. A chemical preservative must be listed by its common name, along with a description of its function, such as "preservative," "a mold inhibitor," or "to promote color retention."

An interesting exception to the rule regarding the order in which ingredients must be listed concerns ingredients that are 2% or less by weight of the food product. Such ingredients may be listed in any order, following the statement "contains less than 2% of ___." It is important to note that this means each single ingredient in the list is less than 2% of the product by weight. Therefore, if there are five ingredients that each comprises 1% of the weight of the product, together they would represent 5% of the product's weight.

Why can producers use the word "or," as when listing the possible oils used? Shouldn't they tell consumers which one was used in the product?

The FDA allows the use of the words and phrases "or," "and/or," and "contains one or more of the following" for food product ingredient lists when "the manufacturer, because of the use of varying mixtures, is unable to adhere to a constant pattern of fats and/or oils in the product." The FDA also permits ingredient names such as "a blend of vegetable oils" when the exact oils used vary or are difficult to specify. It does mandate that all hydrogenated oils be named. But consumers concerned about the types of oils they are consuming may wish to avoid products whose ingredients are unclear. A similar rule applies to other ingredients, such as leavening agents, again when product recipes may vary. An ingredient list may contain a statement such as "contains one or more of the following: baking soda, monocalcium phosphate or calcium carbonate."

30. What are allergens, and what allergens are required to be listed on food labels?

Allergens are substances that cause an allergic response in susceptible people, a type of immune response that, in some cases, can lead to life-threatening symptoms, a condition known as anaphylaxis. For example, people with severe food allergies may experience swelling of the throat and airways when they consume the offending food, making it difficult to breathe. Allergens may be found in many places, including food, medicine, air, fabrics, animals, and plants. The most effective strategy for treating food allergies is to identify and avoid the problematic foods. People who experience severe food allergies must carry medication, usually epinephrine, that is quickly injectable and can help counter the life-threatening symptoms of food allergies.

Food allergies affect about 2% of adults and about 5% of children in the United States. Around 30,000 people are treated in emergency departments each year for food allergies, and 150 people in the United States die each year from allergic reactions to food. The number of people with food allergies has increased significantly over the past decade. For example, peanut allergies have tripled in the past 15 years. It is unclear whether more diagnoses are being made as a result of increased knowledge or as a result of an actual increase in allergy frequency; it is also possible that

some diagnoses are incorrect. Food intolerances affect much larger numbers of people. Prevalence is difficult to estimate, since many people are
never tested and simply avoid certain foods.

A food allergy involves an adverse immune system reaction to a food
or component of food, usually a protein. There are several different ways
in which the immune system can create an allergic response to food molecules. The most dangerous type of food allergy involves the production of
an antibody known as immunoglobulin (IgE). For reasons not yet understood, initial ingestion of the food allergen causes the body to mistakenly produce IgE antibodies to that particular food component. These IgE
antibodies then circulate in the bloodstream and attach to mast cells and
basophils. Mast cells are located in all areas of the body, especially the
respiratory system, the skin, and the gastrointestinal track. Basophils are
found in the blood and in areas inflamed by an allergic reaction. When
the food allergen is subsequently ingested, it binds to the IgE antibodies
that then triggers the mast cells and basophils to release large amounts
of chemicals called histamine. Histamine triggers the inflammation and
swelling associated with an allergic response.

In most cases, an IgE-mediated food allergy will develop within an hour
after eating the food. The consumer will often notice common symptoms:
hives, itching, skin rashes, swelling of the face or throat, wheezing, con-
gestion, trouble breathing, abdominal pain, diarrhea, nausea, vomiting,
dizziness, lightheadedness, and/or fainting. A severe allergic reaction is
called anaphylaxis, and it produces life-threatening signs and symptoms
such as swelling of the throat, shock, drop in blood pressure, irregular or
rapid pulse, and loss of consciousness. Anaphylaxis is potentially fatal.

Less severe food allergies can be mediated by other types of immune
responses. For example, IgG-mediated food allergies tend to develop
more slowly with milder symptoms. IgG-mediated responses may not be
detected with standard diagnostic testing.

To diagnose food allergies, health care providers might use a detailed
history, an oral food challenge, an elimination diet, or skin or blood tests.
The most reliable test for the diagnosis of a food allergy is to observe the
symptoms that develop after a person has consumed a given food. This
test is called an oral food challenge. Patients consume the potentially
problematic food in increasing amounts, and alternating with placebo
components, so that patients do not know when they are consuming
the problem food. (It is possible to experience allergic reactions simply
because one believes one has ingested a certain food, even when the food
has not actually been ingested.) Since patients may develop a severe allergic response, many providers will not administer this test. However, it

is administered in some cases by experienced professionals in an environment that can provide immediate treatment should a severe reaction develop.

Elimination diets can take a variety of forms. The basic goal is to observe a person's response to a diet lacking then later including the potential food allergen. If allergic symptoms go away or do not appear when the food is absent, but appear when the food is added back, providers and patients can discover which foods are problematic. Elimination diets are not recommended for severe allergies but may be helpful for milder food allergy symptoms.

Skin and blood tests measure levels of IgE antibodies but may overdiagnose true allergies. This is because IgE antibodies may be present but not indicate that a patient will develop a full-blown allergic response. Skin tests are rapid and are usually less expensive than a blood test. Two types of skin tests are commonly used: the skin prick test and the intradermal test. The skin prick test is done by adding a drop of the alleged allergen onto the skin's surface which is either scratched or has a series of needle-pricks in it, in order for the solution to enter; if the skin welts, the patient has a positive reaction and is allergic to the allergen. The intradermal test is done when during the skin prick test, the allergen did not test positive but is still thought to be the suspect, because the intradermal test is a much more sensitive test. The allergen is injected right into the skin which is then observed for signs of irritation. The blood tests look for antibodies and are generally performed on patients who can't have skin tests.

The most reliable treatment for suspected food allergies is to avoid problematic foods, hence, the importance of the allergen listing and ingredient lists on food labels.

It is important for people with allergies to be prepared for unexpected exposure: they should wear a medical alert bracelet stating the possibility that they might have a severe allergic reaction, carry an auto-injector device that contains epinephrine, and seek medical help immediately if they experience allergic reactions.

Food allergies are especially prevalent in children; therefore, food allergies are of particular concern in the school environment. Almost 20% of children with food allergies have had allergic reactions after accidentally ingesting a food allergen while in school. Up to 25% of anaphylaxis reactions in school occur in children who were not previously diagnosed with a food allergy. It is vital that school personnel are ready to manage both students with known food allergies and those who have not been diagnosed with any food allergy.

Many people confuse food allergies and food intolerances. Food intolerance symptoms include intestinal gas, abdominal discomfort, diarrhea, hives, headaches, or irritability and usually come on gradually. These symptoms may result from an absence of an enzyme needed to fully digest a food, irritable bowel syndrome, sensitivity to food additives, reoccurring stress, or psychological factors. Food intolerances include reactions to certain products that are added to foods to enhance the taste, add color, or protect against the growth of microbes. Food intolerances can be very uncomfortable, but they are not immediately life-threatening. Because symptoms of food intolerances often overlap with those of food allergies, people who experience such symptoms may benefit from allergy testing to rule out the possibility of a severe reaction. Two of the most common food intolerances include lactose intolerance and celiac disease.

Lactose is a sugar found in milk. Lactase is an enzyme in the lining of the gut that breaks down or digests this lactose; when this enzyme is absent, a person has lactose intolerance. The lactose stays in the digestive tract, producing a variety of digestive symptoms. Once it passes into the colon, it is broken down by bacteria, producing intestinal gas in this fermentation process.

Celiac disease is a food intolerance that elicits a unique physical response. Celiac disease is a condition that is triggered by foods containing gluten, and is present in about 1% of the population. People with celiac disease have an immune system that reacts negatively to the presence of gluten in the diet, but this response is not of the same nature as a typical allergic reaction, in that the immune system attacks the cells lining the small intestine, rather than stimulating anaphylaxis.

Mild forms of food intolerance are often referred to as food sensitivities. People with food sensitivities find that certain foods "disagree" with them. They may feel they have difficulty digesting the food, and they get a stomachache after eating it. For example, people who have been on low-fat diets may find eating a high-fat food such as quiche, french fries, or a fatty burger disagrees with them, feeling heavy and uncomfortable in the stomach. While food sensitivities are milder than food intolerances, food sensitivities can be a real problem for some people.

In 2004, the U.S. Congress passed the Food Allergen Labeling Consumer Protection Act (FALCPA), which went into effect in 2006 in order to protect those with food allergies. The Food and Drug Administration (FDA) is the agency that enforces the Act. Under FALCPA, food labels are required to clearly name major allergens in the list of ingredients. Over 160 foods can cause allergic symptoms in susceptible people.

Obviously, it would be impossible to list all of these on the food label, so FALCPA mandates the listing of the eight foods that account for 90% of all allergens in the United States: milk, eggs, peanuts, tree nuts (e.g., almonds, walnuts, pecans), soybeans, wheat, fish, and crustacean shellfish (e.g., crab, lobster, shrimp). (Molluscan shellfish, such as oysters, clams, mussels, or scallops, are not considered major allergens.) A major food allergen is defined as one of these foods or an ingredient that contains protein derived from one of the allergen food groups.

Major allergens must be identified on the food label in at least one of two ways. Labels may list any of the major eight food allergens contained in the product in a list beneath the ingredients. The statement is in the form "contains _____" with the common name of the allergen(s). Or the common allergen name may be listed in parenthesis in the ingredient list after the ingredient. For example, "lecithin (soy)," "flour (wheat)," and "whey (milk)." Listing the common name is important, since ingredient names may be unfamiliar to some people.

Many food manufacturers add advisory statements to their labels to take into account possible allergen contamination of products because of cross contact, when an allergen not normally present in a food product can become included in the product accidentally. Cross contact may occur during harvesting, transportation, manufacturing, processing, or storage. To account for cross-contamination, labels may now (but are not required to) include advisory statements such as "produced in a plant that processes wheat" or "may have come into contact with nut products." According to the FDA, these advisory statements do not substitute for adhering to current and good manufacturing practices and are required to be truthful and not misleading.

31. What is gluten, and how does a food label get to use a "gluten-free" claim?

Gluten is a protein found in certain grains, including wheat, rye, and barley. People avoid gluten for a variety of reasons. In about 1% of people, gluten elicits an autoimmune response, in which immune cells mistakenly attack the lining of small intestine. People with this autoimmune response and the accompanying damage to the small intestine are diagnosed with celiac disease. Researchers believe that the cause of celiac disease most likely is a combination of genetic and environmental factors. The only treatment for celiac disease is a lifelong gluten-free diet and avoidance of all gluten-containing foods, beverages, and medications, as no cure currently exists for celiac disease. Thus, the labeling of food products is critically important to these individuals and the people who cook for them.

Some people avoid gluten because they are allergic to wheat. A wheat allergy is a type of food allergy. Allergic responses are characterized by a range of symptoms, from hives, rashes, and swelling to difficulty breathing and loss of consciousness. In severe cases, food allergies can be fatal. Wheat allergies are thought to affect about 0.1% of people in North America. Food labeling is critically important to all people with food allergies.

A significant number of people without celiac disease or wheat allergies may experience distressing symptoms, such as intestinal gas, bloating, pain, and constipation, as well as non-gastrointestinal (GI) symptoms such as fatigue and headaches, when they consume gluten-containing foods, a condition known as non-celiac gluten sensitivity (NCGS). To receive a diagnosis of NCGS people must test negatively for celiac disease; experience the functional negative symptoms associated with celiac disease, such as bloating and pain after ingestion of gluten-containing foods; and show symptom improvement with a gluten-free diet. Recent research suggests that many people currently diagnosed or who have self-diagnosed themselves with NCGS may actually be sensitive to food components other than gluten, such as certain types of small carbohydrate groups common in grains. These components have been called "FODMAPs," an acronym that stands for fermentable oligo-, di-, and monosaccharides and polyols. FODMAPs are poorly absorbed in the GI tract of people with functional bowel disorders, such as irritable bowel syndrome. When the FODMAPs reach the large intestine, the microbes living there metabolize these molecules, releasing gas in the process. The gas increases feelings of bloating, pressure, and pain, and may interfere with normal colon motility. The elimination of gluten-containing foods concomitantly reduces intake of these FODMAP components, leading to an amelioration of NCGS symptoms.

People who suspect that they may have a gluten sensitivity of some sort should seek medical advice, and be tested for celiac disease, rather than self-diagnosing this condition. Celiac disease is difficult to diagnose because it is characterized by symptoms that are similar to those of other diseases, such as irritable bowel syndrome or intestinal infections. Symptoms of celiac disease include digestive symptoms such as abdominal bloating and pain, chronic diarrhea, vomiting, constipation, and weight loss. Children with celiac disease may also suffer from irritability, delayed growth, or delayed puberty. Adults often have symptoms that seem unrelated to the digestive system, including iron-deficiency anemia, fatigue, bone or joint pain, arthritis, bone loss or osteoporosis, depression or anxiety, infertility, or skin rashes. Diagnosis is extremely important because celiac disease is a serious illness that can compromise long-term health if untreated. Celiac disease is diagnosed with certain blood tests and usually an intestinal biopsy to check for damage to the intestinal lining.

Gluten-free diets and foods have become popular even among people with no adverse GI reactions to gluten. This may be attributable to popular media that have sensationally painted gluten as a food ingredient responsible for everything from autoimmune diseases to brain disorders such as autism, anxiety, depression, and Alzheimer's disease. While a few research studies have linked gluten consumption to neurological disorders in animals and a small number of humans, especially people with celiac disease, the research is very preliminary at this point. While gluten-free diets have been promoted as successful weight loss strategies, evidence supporting this claim is lacking. Temporary weight loss often occurs when people eliminate foods from their diet. Several studies suggest that gluten and other components of gluten-containing whole grains may have important health benefits for people without celiac disease, wheat allergies, or NCGS, including better colon microbiome composition (beneficial bacteria in the gut) and protection from colon cancer. A diet high in cereal fibers appears to contribute to healthful blood pressure regulation, blood sugar regulation, and blood fat levels. These observations suggest that eliminating wheat, barley, and rye from the diet, in people without celiac disease, wheat allergies, and NCGS, could have negative impacts on public health.

Unless a food is naturally gluten-free (such as, unprocessed fruits, vegetables, and meats), people with celiac disease must assume a food product might contain gluten from some form of contamination, such as that which can occur from food harvesting and storage facilities, or from contact with equipment or surfaces used to process gluten-containing foods, or because the product contains an ingredient containing gluten. The words "gluten-free" on the food label help consumers select products likely to be gluten-free. In addition, people avoiding gluten use the mandatory ingredients list on the food label to search for ingredients that are likely to contain gluten, and avoid products accordingly.

The gluten-free claim on a food label is a voluntary claim; in other words, manufacturers are not required to state whether or not their product contains gluten. This means gluten-free foods are not required to carry the words "gluten-free" on the label. Food products that are labeled gluten-free must meet certain standards. According to Food and Drug Administration (FDA) regulations, a product may claim to be "gluten-free," "without gluten," "no gluten," or "free of gluten" if it has less than 20 parts per million (ppm) of gluten. The FDA permits the manufacturer to place these words anywhere on the label, so long as mandatory labeling requirements are met.

In addition to containing less than 20 ppm of gluten, in order to meet the criteria for a gluten-free label designation, a product must either be inherently gluten-free or does not contain an ingredient that is (1) a gluten-containing grain (e.g., spelt wheat); (2) derived from a gluten-containing grain that has not been processed to remove gluten (e.g., wheat flour); or (3) derived from a gluten-containing grain that has been processed to remove gluten (e.g., wheat starch), if the use of that ingredient results in the presence of 20 parts per million (ppm) or more gluten in the food.

Less than 20 ppm became the allowable level for gluten in gluten-free food because standard methods of chemical analysis in use by food manufacturers at the time of the development of the FDA ruling (2007–2014) could not reliably measure gluten levels below 20 ppm. Twenty ppm means that there are 20 mg of gluten per kilogram of food, or 20 mg of gluten per 35.27 oz of food.

Is less than 20 ppm a safe level of gluten ingestion for people with celiac disease? Scientists believe people with celiac disease vary somewhat in their sensitivity to gluten; therefore, at the present time researchers are unable to establish a level of gluten ingestion that is truly safe for every person with celiac disease. The best diet for people with celiac disease would be one that has a gluten level of 0 ppm. However, some experts have stated that 20 ppm is probably relatively safe for most people with celiac disease. The FDA urges consumers with celiac disease to check with their health care providers for dietary advice on safe levels of gluten ingestion.

Food manufacturers may elect to have their product tested for gluten content levels by third-party (not the FDA and not the manufacturer) gluten-free certification programs. Some of these groups use more specialized equipment that can detect gluten levels below 20 ppm. For example, the Gluten Intolerance Group will certify a product as gluten-free only if gluten levels are at or below 10 ppm. The FDA permits the use of third-party gluten-free logos on food products, providing the food meets the FDA gluten-free standards.

Consumers should note that gluten-free products, such as baked goods, are not automatically healthful foods, but may contain significant amounts of added sugars, salt, and fats.

Other Label Information and Claims

32. Why is country of origin required on some food labels?

A statement declaring the country of origin on a food's label is not required by the Food and Drug Administration (FDA). However, U.S. Customs and Border Protection (CBP) enforces certain labeling requirements in accordance with U.S. and international trade regulations. The CBP is a large federal agency, a part of the Department of Homeland Security, that is charged with safeguarding U.S. borders to protect the public "from dangerous people and materials while enhancing the Nation's global economic competitiveness by enabling legitimate trade and travel." Some of its rules govern food imported from other countries and sold in the United States.

The CBP mandates that companies importing food products include on the food label the English name of the country of origin. Wording for conveying this information is flexible. The label of an olive oil from Spain might carry a country of origin statement such as "country of origin: Spain," or include descriptions such as "Spanish olive oil" or "imported from Spain." Foods sold without packaging, such as fish and shellfish, in a market, may display country of origin on a sign next to the product. On foods governed by the U.S. Department of Agriculture, country of origin may appear on a sign by a product sold without packages, such as fruits and vegetables. Interestingly, as of 2016, beef and pork muscle meat cuts and ground beef and pork do not require country of origin statements, as a result of trade agreements with certain countries.

Sometimes it is not easy to figure out a product's country of origin. In the global marketplace, it is not uncommon for a food to be processed or repackaged in several countries on its way to a store in the United States. For example, nuts harvested in South America might be mixed into a snack bar in a different country, and then imported and repackaged by an importer in the United States. According to the rules of the CBP, if a food undergoes "substantial transformation" at some point in production, that country becomes the "country of origin," no matter where the original food ingredients were grown or produced. Thus, for the snack bar, the country making the nuts into a snack bar would serve as the country of origin.

Rules governing the definition of "substantial transformation" follow the FDA label principle that labels must not be false or misleading. Consider a U.S. company that buys shrimp harvested in another country, and then processes the shrimp by peeling and deveining it, and putting it in a package. The CBP would not consider this "substantial transformation." The package contents would still be labeled "shrimp," and rules would dictate that the original country of origin (where the shrimp was harvested) should be named as country of origin. However, if the shrimp is combined with many other ingredients and made, for example, into frozen stir-fry dinners in the United States, then the United States becomes the country of origin, and the food is no longer required to name the country of origin for the shrimp. A similar situation would be when fresh vegetables grown in several countries are imported and made into a frozen mixed vegetable product in the United States. Since the mixing and freezing of the vegetables would not qualify as "substantial transformation," the product should be labeled with the country of origin for each ingredient. However, if the vegetables were used to create a canned soup with many additional ingredients in the United States, the United States becomes the country of origin, and the label would not need a country of origin statement.

Country of origin statements sometimes name the different countries involved in producing a product. For example, a can of tuna fish might declare something like: "Caught in Pacific Ocean. Product of China. Canned in the U.S."

Understanding country of origin regulations helps consumers see that label statements such as "American Made" may not reveal much about the origin of the ingredients in products that combine (and sub-stantially transform) multiple ingredients. Some people would like more information about product components. They may not trust or wish to support agricultural practices in certain countries, being con-cerned, for example, about the use of certain pesticides, or about animal care regulations. Some consumers may wish to boycott a given product from a specific country or countries because the consumers are opposed to the working conditions of the people who raise or process the food. And others are concerned about the environmental impact of the prod-ucts they purchase, aware that transporting food long distances gener-ates more greenhouse gases, preferring to buy from local sources when possible.

33. What are nutrient content claims, and what do they mean?

Nutrient content claims are statements regarding the amount of a nutri-ent in a food product. These claims are regulated by the Food and Drug Administration (FDA) and the U.S. Department of Agriculture (USDA) so that all food labels are using the same standard. Therefore, the claims such as "low sodium" carry the same meaning from product to product.

Food packages have carried various statements about their products' nutritive quality, probably for as long as labels have been in existence. These statements are designed to appeal to health-conscious consumers and increase product desirability. Nutrient content claims such "low fat" and "high fiber" proliferated on labels with little regulation during the 1970s and 1980s as people became more aware of the link between diet and health. The dramatic increase in label claims, the meanings of which were unclear and which varied from product to product, prompted the FDA to regulate these claims with the passage of the Nutrition Labeling and Education Act in 1990.

The FDA regulates nutrient content claims for three reasons. First, the FDA hopes that nutrient content claims on food packages will help con-sumers make good food choices to improve their diets. Second, the FDA regulates claims to reduce confusion: it wants consumers to be confident in the meaning of nutrient content statements. Its goal is to create nutri-ent content claims that reflect dietary guidelines such as those from the Department of Health and Human Services. And lastly, the FDA hopes that by allowing and regulating nutrient content claims, manufacturers and food producers will be encouraged to develop and market healthful food products that will appeal to consumers.

Food producers preparing to release a new product must notify the FDA of nutrient content claims they are planning to display on the new food's label 120 days before the product is introduced into the market. Various private agencies, food testing labs, and software programs can help a manufacturer identify which nutrient content claims the new food is eligible to display. Nutrient content claims are based on the percentage of a nutrient's Daily Value contained in one serving of the food. In general, the following terminology is used.

- "Free": The food contains the lowest possible amount of the nutrient per serving.
- "Very low" and "low": The food has some of that nutrient, but at fairly low values.
- "Reduced," "less," or "fewer": The food contains at least 25% less of the nutrient per serving than the usual product.
- "More" and "good source of": The food has at least 10% of the Daily Value per serving for a particular nutrient.
- "High in": The food provides 20% or more of the Daily Value of that nutrient.

Other common regulated nutrient content claims and terminology include the following:

- "Fortified" and "enriched": Vitamins and/or minerals have been added to the food product so that the product offers at least 10% more of the nutrient(s) than are normally found in such products. "Fortified" is used to describe nutrients normally found in the food but are lost during processing, such as B vitamins that are lost when wheat is made into white flour. "Enriched" refers to nutrients not normally found in the food but are added to the product.
- "Light" or "lite": These descriptors can refer to fat, calorie, or sodium content of a food. When referring to fat and/or calories, the terms mean that the food has at least 50% less fat than the regular product. If less than 50% of the calories in that product are from fat, then "light" and "lite" mean that the product contains at least one-third fewer calories. When a label states "light (lite) in sodium," the food must have at least 50% less sodium than the regular product.
- "Lean" and "extra lean": These terms are regulated by the USDA for meat and poultry products. "Lean" means the food provides less than

10 g of fat, 4.5 g of saturated fat, and 95 mg of cholesterol per serving. "Extra lean" denotes less than 5 g of fat, 2 g of saturated fat, and 96 mg of cholesterol per serving.

Consumers can always check the Nutrition Facts panel on a food product to find more precise values for nutrients they are interested in. Even nutrients not normally required on the Nutrition Facts panel must be listed if a label claim is made. For example, if a label states "high in magnesium," then the amount of magnesium per serving, along with the % Daily Value that amount represents, must appear on the Nutrition Facts panel.

34. What health claims are allowed on food labels, and who decides whether a product label can include that claim?

Health claims are statements regarding the association between specific foods or food components and reduced risk of a particular disease or health problem. These claims are regulated by the Food and Drug Administration (FDA) primarily to prevent food producers from exaggerating the potential health benefits of their products. Food producers must submit the health claims they plan to use on their food labels and the nutrition information of their product to the FDA for review before the food is put on the market.

Health claims must be limited to statements about "risk reduction" and may not state that the food or food component can help diagnose, cure, lessen, or treat a disease or health problem. All claims must include the word "may" or "might," so as to not overstate the associations between foods and the prevention of health problems. For example, an allowable health claim can include wording to the effect that a diet with enough calcium and vitamin D may reduce risk of osteoporosis.

The FDA allows two types of health claims on food packages: authorized health claims and qualified health claims. Authorized health claims are statements that, according to the FDA, are supported by significant scientific agreement of qualified experts that the scientific evidence for a substance-disease relationship is very strong. Authorized health claims are typically based on hundreds of scientific studies and extensive analysis by health experts. As new scientific evidence becomes available, the FDA monitors whether or not authorized health claims should be allowed or changed. For example, in 2017 the FDA began to study whether or not the evidence linking soy protein to decreased risk of cardiovascular disease was strong enough to allow food producers to use a health claim to this effect.

Qualified health claims are backed by some scientific evidence but do not meet the criteria for "significant scientific agreement" required for authorized health claims. Interestingly, qualified health claims were created in 1999 in response to the pressure from food and supplement manufacturers. The court ruled in the manufacturers' favor, allowing them to exercise their constitutional right to free speech, claiming to provide consumers with information from "emerging science." While many public health experts feared a proliferation of qualified health claims on food labels following the creation of qualified health claims, this has not become the case. Instead, most manufacturers have opted for structure-function claims (see Question 35).

Products featuring qualified health claims must also include some sort of disclaimer explaining that the scientific evidence supporting the claim is limited. For example, the FDA would allow the following qualified health claim: "Scientific evidence suggests, but does not prove, that whole grains (three servings or 48 g per day), as part of a low saturated fat, low cholesterol diet, may reduce the risk of diabetes mellitus type 2."

Health claim statements must reflect the idea that it is a diet or eating pattern high in the given component that is associated with risk reduction, rather than consumption of a specific food or food product. This specification is very important scientifically, as evidence regarding the links between diet and health reflects overall dietary patterns rather than associations between individual foods and risk reduction. In addition, public health experts emphasize the importance of urging people to develop healthy eating patterns, rather than focusing too much advice on individual foods or food components, which can quickly become very confusing and misleading.

Food producers must study the extensive FDA regulations for each health claim they hope to use on their packaging and conform to all requirements. Consider the example of a producer of muffins high in oat bran fiber, hoping to use a health claim that diets rich in certain types of fiber reduce risk of cardiovascular disease. In addition to meeting the FDA's requirement for the amount of oat bran fiber per serving, the muffins must not exceed specific limits for saturated fat, cholesterol, or sodium per serving. These additional criteria help to prevent products that are generally not so healthful from making health claims based on the presence of one helpful ingredient.

The FDA allows food producers to petition the FDA to use a new health claim. The process is extensive and includes following the FDA guidelines for such petitions and supplying summaries of the scientific evidence supporting the claim. This means that health claims, especially qualified health claims, may be added or deleted as the FDA sees fit.

The authorized health claims consumers are most likely to see on food labels include the following dietary pattern and disease risk associations:

- Diets with adequate calcium and vitamin D and a reduced risk of osteoporosis
- Low intakes of saturated fat and cholesterol and a reduced risk of cardiovascular disease
- Diets rich in fruits, vegetables, and grain products that contain fiber and a reduced risk of cardiovascular disease
- Diets high in fatty acids from oils present in fish and a lower risk of cardiovascular disease
- Diets rich in whole grain foods and other plant foods, as well as low in total fat, saturated fat, and cholesterol, and a reduced risk of cardiovascular disease and certain cancers
- Dietary patterns low in sodium and high in potassium and reduced risk of hypertension and stroke
- Diets low in total fat and a reduced risk of some cancers
- Diets high in fiber, containing grain products, fruits, and vegetables, and lower risk of some cancers
- High intakes of fruits and vegetables and a reduced risk of some cancers
- Adequate intake of folic acid and reduced risk of neural tube defects (a type of birth defect)
- Sugarless gum and reduced risk of tooth decay

35. What are structure/function claims?

Structure/function claims are statements that describe possible effects of a food, food component, or dietary supplement component on body structures or functions, such as bone health, digestion, or immune system function. The rules for using structure/function claims differ slightly between conventional foods and dietary supplements. The Food and Drug Administration (FDA) goal for both, however, is that claims do not imply that the effects are those of a drug, as drugs are regulated differently by the FDA. Structure/function claims may say that foods support health, but not make claims that the food can treat or cure a disease. For example, a beverage enriched with certain nutrients might claim "strengthens the immune system," but it may not say "prevents colds." According to the FDA, the claims for foods must be related to a food's nutritive value. Dietary supplements may claim that the supplement components have certain healthful effects but must be accompanied by the disclaimer "These statements have not been evaluated by the Food and Drug Administration. This product is not intended to diagnose, treat, cure or prevent any disease."

Structure/function claims are permitted to link a nutrient to prevention of an established nutrient deficiency disease ("Vitamin C prevents scurvy"), but then must state the prevalence of the disease in the United States. Since nutrient deficiency diseases are not widespread in the United States (with the exception of iron-deficiency anemia), these claims are not common. Instead, most structure/function claims are statements that describe the way in which a nutrient helps maintain normal structure or function. Wording of these claims varies and is not prescribed by the FDA. Typical claims include "calcium builds strong bones," "fiber maintains bowel regularity," and "antioxidants maintain cell integrity."

Manufacturers whose labels make structure/function claims are supposed to have reliable scientific evidence that their claims are accurate and not misleading, but they are not required to submit this information to the FDA before marketing the product. This means that the FDA does not oversee or approve these claims before a product goes to market. If the FDA is made aware of inappropriate claims once the product is on the market, it can fine the offending manufacturer and require the product be withdrawn from the market, which is very expensive for the manufacturer. Nevertheless, misleading claims do sometimes appear, and not all offending labels are caught.

Many government, public health, and consumer groups have expressed concern that some structure/function claims appearing on food labels may be misleading and lack scientific support. Studies have found some claims appearing on labels imply that the product helps to prevent or treat disease, which is not permitted in a structure/function claim. These studies have found that some companies do not notify the FDA properly regarding their claims. Consumers should therefore be somewhat wary of structure/function claims, and take them with a grain of salt.

36. What does the wording "USDA Organic" on a food label indicate?

The wording "USDA Organic" on a food label indicates that the food has been produced in accordance with rules established by the U.S. Department of Agriculture's (USDA's) National Organics Program (NOP). With the exception of foods produced on very small farms, only products that have been certified by the NOP may use the word "organic" on food labels in the United States. The NOP regulates the term "organic" so that consumers can be assured that the term has meaning, and that food products displaying the term on food labels are made with ingredients, or are themselves foods, produced on farms actually using organic farming methods, as defined by the USDA.

The NOP evolved in response to consumer concerns about farming methods that damage the environment and produce food that may contain chemicals harmful to health. According to the USDA, livestock and agricultural products certified as "USDA Organic" have been produced "without synthetic fertilizers, sewage sludge, irradiation, or genetic engineering." Producers have used farming methods that "maintain or enhance soil and water quality while conserving wetlands, woodlands, and wildlife."

The NOP was first established in the 1990 Farm Bill, in a provision called the Organic Foods Production Act. The USDA's NOP is overseen by a branch of the USDA called the Agricultural Marketing Service. Farmers can obtain the USDA Organic certification for their products by applying to the USDA. As part of the certification process, the farm is visited by an agent certified by the USDA, who inspects the farm to be sure the NOP guidelines are being followed. Farmers must pay an application fee and a fee for the inspection. They must also pay an annual certification fee. This process can cost several hundred dollars, which is why small farms are exempt. It's important to note, however, that small farms are very small, defined as those that produce less than $5,000 of gross income per year. These businesses are most likely to sell their products at their farms or at local farmers markets. Any other producer who has not been certified but uses the word "organic" on a food label may be fined by the USDA.

The USDA's website spells out in great detail exactly what chemicals and other agents are permitted in crop production and the raising of livestock. (In fact, since the creation of the NOP, a small number of synthetic pesticides have been approved and are permitted. These are clearly listed on the NOP's website. They have been determined to not harm human health or the environment.) The NOP also describes how organic products must be processed and stored in order to maintain the organic certification. For example, producers must avoid mixing between organic and nonorganic produce. Only certain chemicals are allowed as sanitizers on processing equipment. And only small amounts of certain non-organic ingredients may be added to organic foods during processing. Meat and meat products certified as USDA Organic must come from animals that have access to the outdoors; are not given antibiotics, growth hormones, or other drugs to prevent disease; and are fed organic feed.

The USDA permits three label statements with the word "organic."

- Labels stating "100% organic" must include only certified organic ingredients in the product. These items may display the USDA Organic Seal on the food package.
- Labels simply claiming "organic" must have at least 95% certified organic ingredients and may include the USDA Organic Seal on the package.
- A label may state "made with organic ingredients" if at least 70% of the ingredients are certified organic. However, these products may not display the USDA Organic Seal on product packages.

37. How are label claims about animal treatment regulated?

Many consumers are concerned about methods used in the raising and slaughtering of livestock. Some are concerned because of their belief that animals should be treated as humanely as possible. Animal treatment also impacts the environment. For example, confined animal feeding operations, where animals spend all of their time in a small indoor area, can damage water quality of that farming community and surrounding area. Animal rearing methods also affect the nutritive quality of the animal product consumed. Studies have found that meat from ruminants such as cattle fed solely on grass differs in fat composition from animals whose feed includes grain, with meat from grass-fed animals containing higher percentages of helpful omega-3 fatty acids.

In an effort to address these concerns, manufacturers of meat, dairy, and egg products use many terms to try to convince consumers that animals have been treated humanely. Some of the terminology and practices are somewhat regulated by the U.S. Department of Agriculture (USDA). While the USDA does have some basic standards for livestock rearing, it generally does not inspect farms to evaluate humane treatment claims. Label terminology defined by the USDA includes the following:

- "Natural": The USDA requires that meat and poultry producers using the word "natural" on their label must show that the product does not contain artificial flavoring, chemical preservatives, or coloring ingredients, and has only been minimally processed. Consumers should also note that while the Food and Drug Administration (FDA) does not strictly regulate this term on the labels it oversees, it does mandate that use of the word "natural" must not be misleading. Therefore, the FDA states that foods labeled as natural should not contain artificial or synthetic additives, such as colors, flavors, and preservatives. This term is relatively meaningless, however, since definitions of natural vary greatly from one label to the next, and no third-party verifications for the term exist.
- "No added hormones": The USDA only allows hormone use in beef cattle and lamb production. (These may not be certified organic.) If a USDA-inspected producer wishes to use the term "no added hormones" on their label, the producer must keep records documenting that no hormones were given to the animals.
- "Grass fed": To use this term on the label, a USDA-inspected producer must keep records documenting that the animals received a majority of their nutrients from grass. The designation "grass fed" on a USDA label does not mean that the products are organic or that the animal was fed only grass.
- "Free range/free roaming": While this term, typically applied to chickens laying eggs, is not strictly defined by the USDA, USDA-inspected producers may use this term if they can document that the animals were sheltered in an area with unlimited access to food and fresh water, and continuous outdoor access, which can mean simply that the building has a small concrete porch.
- "Cage free": Like free range, this term is not defined by the USDA. But producers may use the term on egg cartons if they can document the claim. Cage free indicates that the poultry were able to move freely in their area with unlimited access to food and water.

In addition to the USDA, several third-party organizations have evolved to define and verify livestock husbandry practices. (A third-party organization comprises neither governmental officials nor producers.) These

third-party organizations have more specific criteria for animal treatment and perform farm inspections. Their animal treatment requirements are generally more stringent than the USDA's, and because they
actually do farm inspections, their labels are more meaningful. They
each have their own special seals and label claims that may appear on
food labels for eggs, dairy, and meat products. How trustworthy are these
certifications? These third-party organizations have in turn been evaluated by a highly respected consumer advocacy group, Consumers Union.
Consumers Union is an independent nonprofit organization, with no
financial ties to food producers, governmental organizations such as
the FDA or USDA, or the third-party organizations that inspect and
verify animal treatment practices on farms. Some of the third-party
verifications that appear on food labels, claiming humane treatment of
livestock, that have been evaluated by Consumers Union include the
following:

- "Animal Welfare Approved": This verification seal receives very high
  ratings from Consumers Union. Products displaying this seal on the
  label come from animals raised on farms where they can roam on pasture and have enough space to engage in their normal behaviors. For
  example, chickens are able to scratch and peck the ground.
- "Certified Humane": This verification program also receives high ratings from Consumers Union, although in some areas it is not quite
  as strict as Animal Welfare Approved. Consumers can trust product
  label claims, such as "free range" and "pasture raised" when this seal is
  on the food label.
- "Global Animal Partnership": This program was established by Whole
  Foods for its meat product suppliers. The Global Animal Partnership
  program has six rating levels, with Step 1 being the most basic (similar to traditional agricultural livestock rearing practices) and Step 5+
  being the most humane.
- "American Humane Certified": Rated by Consumers Union as less
  strict in some areas, but when combined with the claim "free range"
  or "pasture raised," people can be confident that the claims are
  meaningful.

Some label claims are for specific issues only. For example, the "American
Grassfed" label is highly meaningful, and consumers can be confident that
this label indicates animals have had only grass in their diets (after wean-
ing). Grain feed is prohibited, as are animal byproducts, antibiotics, and
growth hormones. Animals are treated humanely, and farmers manage

pasture and other lands sustainably. The same is true for the "Certified Grassfed by AGW" label. (AGW stands for "A Greener World," a certifying organization.) "PCO Certified 100% GrassFed" is also a reliable label (PCO stands for Pennsylvania Certified Organic), according to Consumers Union.

38. What are GMOs, and what are the labeling rules for GMO foods or food products made with GMO ingredients?

Genetically modified organisms (GMOs) are plants and animals whose genetic material has been altered using genetic engineering techniques. While people have been genetically modifying food for centuries through cross-pollination, grafting, and other forms of cross breeding, biotechnology experts have developed tools that allow them to alter an organism's genetic makeup with more precision, even inserting genes not naturally found in the target organism. The goal of genetic modification is to improve an organism, for example, making a plant more resistant to disease or drought. Opponents of genetic modification worry that the long-term safety of these procedures is unknown, in terms of impact on the consumer in the case of genetically modified food, or the environment.

To create a food, such as a tomato, using a more traditional breeding technique, the DNA from one type of tomato is crossed with the DNA from another type via pollination, with the hopes of creating a plant with desired traits, such as increased sweetness, pest resistance, or more durability for the long journey to the supermarket. However, this process transfers both desired and undesired genes, so it can take many generations before the ideal traits are achieved, if at all. Biotechnology offers a more precise way to modify an organism's DNA. Recombinant DNA biotechnology allows scientists to take a specific piece of DNA from one plant or animal and combine it with a strand of DNA from another plant or animal. Instead of sharing thousands of genes (as with traditional breeding), genetic engineering allows a single gene to be exchanged. It also allows for combinations of DNA from organisms never before possible. Newer gene-editing techniques such as CRISPR (clustered regularly interspersed short palindromic repeats) have created a variety of food products and food production techniques.

The Flavr Savr tomato was the world's first commercially available "genetically modified" food and was introduced to consumers in supermarkets in 1994. It did not prove to be profitable, but it opened the door to a new era of food production. With its advent arose enormous questions of how, why, and when to use GMOs, and whether these foods require special labeling.

The United States is the largest producer of GM crops. Over 90 percent of all cotton and soybeans planted in the United States are genetically engineered, as well as 88 percent of corn. Other common GM crops include canola, alfalfa, and sugar beets. Most of these crops are engineered to tolerate herbicide or fight off pests. For example, Roundup Ready soybeans are tolerant to the herbicide glyphosate (both products are produced by the same corporation, Monsanto). Other crops, such as Bt corn, contain DNA from a microorganism, *Bacillus thuringiensis* (Bt), that produces chemicals toxic to insects. Bt corn, therefore, produces its own insecticide against the European corn borer insect.

The major GM crops are used to produce animal feed and food ingredients, such as corn starch, corn syrup, cottonseed oil, soybean oil, and canola oil. These ingredients are then used to make soups, salad dressings, cereals, chips, and other processed foods. Whole foods such as fruits and vegetables are less commonly made with genetic engineering, although that may change with increased consumer support. The Food and Drug Administration (FDA) approved the marketing of GM salmon in March 2019, engineered to grow more quickly than normal salmon.

Gene editing has proven to be especially useful for manufacturing a variety of enzymes, flavors, and other additives used in food processing. For example, cheese makers use an enzyme called chymosin to turn milk into cheese; chymosin drives the milk-curdling process. About 90 percent of the cheeses produced in the United States use a chymosin produced by a genetically engineered bacterium. This chymosin is chemically identical to traditionally produced chymosin, which is taken from the stomach lining of unweaned calves, a much more expensive process.

Debate over GMOs frequently focuses on its regulation, which varies widely from country to country, and even from state to state within the United States because of new food labeling initiatives. In the United States, three federal agencies work in conjunction to regulate GMOs: the FDA, which is responsible for ensuring the safety of human and animal food; the U.S. Department of Agriculture (USDA), which is responsible for protecting agriculture from pest and disease; and the Environmental Protection Agency, which regulates food safety when connected with environmental concerns, such as pesticide use and crops that are genetically engineered to create their own pesticide, such as Bt corn. GM foods must meet the same safety standards as traditional foods, as well as undergo tests for potential new toxins and allergens and any long-term risks from consumption. Nutrient levels between the GM crop and traditional crop are also compared.

Whether and how to label GMO foods and foods produced with GMO ingredients is a contentious issue. While consumer groups claim people have a right to know how their food is produced and what ingredients are in a food product, industry and many scientific groups believe consumers lack the education to understand genetic engineering. The first U.S. regulation regarding labeling of GMO products came in the form of a policy statement by the FDA. The FDA ruled that GMO foods only needed to be labeled as such if materially different from conventional counterparts. This rule was hard to interpret and produced a great deal of confusion for food producers and consumers alike. When the USDA created its National Organic Program, it mandated no GMO ingredients in foods labeled USDA Organic. Other organic labels have followed suit.

Many states dissatisfied with the FDA ruling have been discussing GMO labeling issues for years, with Vermont becoming the first state to mandate the labeling of GMO foods in 2016. In the same year, the U.S. Congress passed a bill requiring GMO labeling on food labels. However, much to the chagrin of many consumer rights' groups, such labeling can be provided through label text, a symbol, a toll-free number, or simply a QR code consumers can access with a smart phone to get more information. Many people do not have smart phones or reliable Internet connections. It also seems unlikely that shoppers will take time in the supermarket to use their phones to research the products they are considering buying.

Consumers who wish to avoid GMO foods can look for foods labeled USDA Organic, as well as many other organic labels. For example, the "Organic is always nonGMO" label from Organic Valley and Organic Prairie brands conforms to USDA organic standards, not allowing GMO ingredients. Other trustworthy organic/non-GMO labels include those from California Certified Organic Farmers and the Northeast Organic Farming Association. The Non-GMO Project Verified label has received high marks from independent evaluator Consumers Union. All products with the Non-GMO Project Verified label meet the Project's standards, certified to contain no GMO ingredients.

Case Studies

1. TRACKING NUTRIENTS TO IMPROVE SPORT PERFORMANCE

Lauren's second year as a defender on her college soccer team was marked by inconsistent performance. Some matches were awesome: she intercepted balls from the opposing strikers, worked well with the other defenders to block shots on goal, and had plenty of energy to follow the directions of the center defender. But sometimes she had trouble keeping her head in the game. She felt tired, had trouble focusing, and spent much of these games on the bench.

At the end of the season, Lauren's coach met with her, and they discussed her performance. Lauren was excited to hear that she was being considered to serve as a center defender next year, since the players currently holding that position were graduating. However, the coach emphasized that Lauren needed to spend more of her time playing at her best. Lauren and the coach explored factors that might be holding her back. The coach suggested Lauren work hard during the off season on her nutrition and fitness to see if improving these might boost her performance. She referred Lauren to the campus sport nutritionist and encouraged her to do her best as the team worked with the strength and conditioning coach.

Lauren suspected the coach was on the right track. Lauren began playing soccer in middle school to lose weight. Her strong, muscular body would never be that of the current fashion model build, but she had tried to achieve this body type nevertheless. Throughout the years, she had followed every diet imaginable, losing and regaining the same 10 or 15 lbs over and over. This past year she had tried limiting carbohydrate foods and eating more protein, thinking that might give her more energy.

"Wrong approach," declared the sport nutritionist. "No wonder you are having problems on the field. You need to do a better job of fueling your body." Lauren's body composition was not too bad, and in her discussions with the nutritionist she began to understand she could struggle forever to try to make her body something it wasn't, or she could embrace her athletic potential and eat to win. The nutritionist had Lauren download an app for her smartphone that would help her track her macros—fat, protein, and carbohydrate—each day. The nutritionist gave her target ranges for these that would result in a more balanced nutrient intake. They made general meal plan guidelines for Lauren to follow, based on foods Lauren liked to eat that were accessible to her. Lauren's nutritionist never used the word "diet" but always referred to Lauren's guidelines as her sport training eating plan.

Lauren was also in the weight room several times a week lifting with her team. Her goals were to increase her strength and speed. Her body responded well to the work. Gaining weight was a little scary, but her nutritionist kept track of her body composition and assured Lauren she was actually gaining muscle, not fat. Training with her team was fun—there was always great music in the weight room, and as Lauren's strength improved, she was motivated to continue her training and her eating plan.

The phone app kept track of nutrients using the food bar codes as well as data Lauren entered regarding portion sizes. Lauren was already pretty much of an expert at reading food labels, and using them to track her training diet was not hard. Since she usually had her phone with her, entering foods as she ate them was convenient. Each week, she shared her data with her nutritionist. This motivated Lauren to stick with the program. Some weeks, her macros were adjusted if she was gaining fat, or if her energy level was low.

The food labels also provided information on a variety of nutrients, and the nutritionist pointed out to Lauren that her vitamin and mineral intakes were improving with the new meal plan. Her iron and calcium were right on target, as was vitamin D. Her potassium intake was always a little below the recommended daily value, although it increased as Lauren added more vegetables to her lunch and dinner choices. Her nutritionist emphasized the importance of improving potassium intake, as this mineral is important for muscle function.

Being able to track her nutrients throughout the day helped guide Lauren's food choices at meal time. If she noticed she was falling behind on carbohydrates, for example, she would add more carbohydrate-rich choices to her next meal or snack. For Lauren, using food labels with a nutrient-tracker app encouraged healthful food choices. After a few weeks, she settled into a fairly routine eating pattern that provided the fuel she needed for her sport training. Not only was she getting stronger and faster, but she also had more energy throughout the day and found both her training and schoolwork easier.

Analysis

Not so long ago, tracking nutrient intake was painstakingly time consuming. Entering a day's worth of food consumption into a computer program could be boring at best, difficult and frustrating at worst. With the advent of smartphone apps that can quickly access data from food labels, logging meals and snacks has become much easier. (Some apps even provide data from a photo of the food on one's plate.)

Many studies have found that self-monitoring reinforces behavior change goals and increases the likelihood of success in behavior change programs. Interestingly, the accuracy of the values recorded bears little relationship to behavior change success. For people using food labels, the fact that food label values can be 20% higher or lower than what the labeled food contains is irrelevant, even in terms of calorie counts. In the long run, it all evens out, and people do well with their eating plans, as illustrated by Lauren's example.

Caution: People with certain types of eating disorders and disordered eating behaviors should not monitor food intake. Some people with eating disorders are already too compulsive about monitoring their diets; using the smartphone apps only worsens their disorders and interferes with recovery.

2. CHOOSING HEALTHY FOODS ON A BUDGET

Lee is a college sophomore, majoring in economics and serving as coeditor for the student newspaper. Last year he lived in the dorms and had to participate in the college's dining system, which seemed very expensive to him. He figured he could save a bucket of money by moving off campus and eating on his own. Lee and three of his friends found an apartment not too far from campus and began sophomore year treasuring their independence and counting all the money they would save by not paying for the college's meal plan.

Lee and his friends had very different schedules between their classes, activities, and part-time jobs, so they decided not to try to coordinate and share meals together. Instead, they decided that each person would take care of his own food needs. Lee was no stranger to the aisles of the grocery store, but he had never shopped regularly before. At the beginning of the year, he loaded up his cart with cheap food that was easy to prepare. He bought oatmeal for breakfast—he could buy huge containers so the cereal was only pennies per serving. Lunch would be peanut butter sandwiches. Dinner would be pasta and sauce, macaroni and cheese, canned soup, or ramen noodles. Lee used the product price comparison information on the grocery shelves to choose the cheapest products and stretch his food dollar as far as possible.

The beginning of the school year was exciting. Lee enjoyed settling into his classes and getting the school paper up and running again. Lee's food plan seemed to work well at first. The food required little time to prepare, and cleanup was not too bad. But after a few weeks Lee became pretty bored with the monotony of his meals. He also felt hungry in the late afternoons, so he would grab a snack (usually the cheapest choices: potato chips or cookies) from the vending machines near the school paper office. In the evenings he and his roommates would often order pizza (plain cheese, the cheapest choice and lots of it) to sustain them through their study (and video game) sessions.

After midterms, Lee came down with one cold after another. He felt tired all the time, and the waist on his pants was feeling tight. When his roommate was diagnosed with mono, Lee went to health services to get tested as well. Thankfully, he tested negative, but the kind nurse sat him down and started asking him questions about his lifestyle. As they discussed his eating habits, she started taking a lot of notes. At the end of the appointment, she printed out some simple meal guidelines from the MyPlate website and told Lee he needed to increase his intake of fruits and vegetables, take a multivitamin and mineral supplement, and be sure he was getting enough protein. She told him for a man of his size, 180 lbs, he should be getting at least 65 g of protein a day. Since he had gained 10 lbs since the beginning of the semester she advised him to cut back on the refined carbohydrates (pasta, bread) and choose foods with greater nutrient density, more nutrition per calorie.

Lee decided to track his protein intake. He checked the food labels of his staples. Didn't the chicken noodle soup have more protein?

Only 3 g per serving. Wasn't that can two servings? Lee read the nutrition facts panel more closely. Oh, the entire can was 2.5 servings, so he was getting 7.5 g, since he usually consumed the whole can. What about the peanut butter? Seven grams of protein per 2 tablespoon serving. What exactly is a tablespoon? Lee wondered. Was he even using 2 tablespoons per day? Ramen noodles? 4.5 g per serving. Thank goodness for the milk he poured on his oatmeal: 8 g per cup. Hmmm, did he use a whole cup? Oatmeal contributed about 6 g per cup. Lee added up his protein intake:

Oatmeal	6 g
Milk	8 g
Peanut butter	7 g
Bread	6 g
Soup	4–7 g (depending on choice of soup)

Lee was alarmed to see that some days he was only getting about 34 g of protein a day, far short of the 65 g recommended by the nurse. Thankfully, that cheese pizza added 12 g/slice. But after taking a look at the labels on his food staples, Lee was forced to conclude that his diet probably lacked not only protein but many vitamins and minerals as well.

Analysis

It is not uncommon for busy people living on their own for the first time to have some difficulties figuring out how to shop for food and prepare meals on a budget. Many people find that food labels can be a good place to start. The information presented on food labels is easily accessible and provides the basics for many important nutrients. People new to shopping and cooking are likely to rely more heavily on the packaged food that carry food labels than people who prepare their own meals from nonlabeled foods such as vegetables and fruits.

Lee is typical of many people living in the United States in that he expects to be able to spend relatively little money on food. People in the United States spend the lowest percentage of their income on food of any other country in the world—a little over 6% on average. Grocery stores and restaurant chains cater to people who tend to shop by price rather than nutritive value or gastronomic quality. People like Lee often search for ways to get the most food for the least amount of money because of financial constraints. But the cheapest packaged foods tend to be lower in protein and other important nutrients. Over time, poor nutrition can lead to health problems, such as those experienced by Lee: a lowered resistance to colds and flus.

Developing good eating habits takes time and knowledge, especially when one is shopping for and preparing meals with a limited budget. The U.S. Department of Agriculture's (USDA's) choosemyplate website (https://www.choosemyplate.gov/budget) is a good place to start. It offers many good suggestions for healthy eating when the cost of food is an important consideration.

3. USING FOOD LABELS TO PREVENT CHRONIC DISEASE

Jessica's grandmother started dialysis when Jessica was only 12. Her grandmother's failing kidneys were no longer doing an adequate job of purifying her blood, due to her type 2 diabetes. Jessica learned that diabetes means high blood sugar levels that harm the blood vessels and organs of the body. Jessica's grandmother lived next door, and Jessica's family helped to take care of her. In fact, Jessica's mom had to cut back her work hours once Jessica's grandmother needed dialysis. Dialysis treatments take a long time—several hours, and Jessica's mom couldn't manage both full-time work and care of her mother.

Jessica was worried, because she knew her mother also had diabetes. "Are my mom's kidneys going to fail too? And what about me?" Jessica wondered. "Is diabetes something everyone in my family has to get?"

Four year later, Jessica learned in her high school health class that type 2 diabetes was very common and was often caused by obesity, especially excess body fat in the abdominal area. There was a genetic component as well—it did run in families. Everyone is Jessica's family was fairly overweight. Her mother and father were both rather short and round, as were her grandparents. She herself was short, but she had a lovely figure, as her mother would say. Jessica was much more active than her parents and enjoyed the dance classes at her school. But what would happen as she got older?

Jessica decided to talk to her health teacher to learn more about diabetes and whether or not it could be prevented. She was happy to learn there was a good chance of preventing, or at least significantly delaying, the development of diabetes with a healthy lifestyle. The health teacher encouraged Jessica to stay active and have a healthy diet. A healthy diet was one with lots of fruits and vegetables, but low in food products with added sugars. Jessica registered for the health teacher's nutrition course the following semester, to learn more about eating well and preventing diabetes.

Added sugars. Jessica knew reducing added sugars was not going to be easy for her or her mom. Jessica's mom loved to bake, and the family enjoyed dessert after dinner every night. Dinner itself was often sweet: brown sugar on the squash, barbecue sauce on the meat, marshmallows on the sweet potatoes. Large bottles of soda accompanied salty snacks throughout the day.

At the beginning of the next semester, Jessica had to record and analyze her food intake for three days for her nutrition class. What an eye-opening exercise! As expected, her added sugars were very high, and the computer program the class used helped her see where these were in her diet: everywhere.

Jessica became an avid food label reader. She found that a 20 fluid ounce bottle of soda had 65 g of added sugar—130% of the Daily Value! But she loved soda. Jessica decided she would try to learn to like diet soda—or maybe try mixing fruit juice with seltzer. That might not be too bad.

What to do about the sugar in the family meals and in the house? Jessica was not sure how much dietary change her family could take. Her mother was busier than ever these days, so Jessica hated to place more demands on her. She offered to help her mother with grocery shopping and dinner preparation. Her mother loved this idea! The two worked together to plan the following week's meals and a grocery list.

As she shopped for her family, Jessica spent a lot of time reading labels and comparing products. She was surprised to find so much sugar in so many food products. Even some brands of chicken soup had sugar added! Over time, she learned which brands of the foods her family used had less sugar or no sugar added.

Over time, Jessica took over more of the meal planning, gradually replacing sugar-sweetened recipes with interesting alternatives. She started trying new recipes and experimenting with different herbs and spices. Not every meal was a success, but her family members were good sports, and only her little brother complained. Jessica began eating smaller portions of desserts and continued to cut down on soda and sugary snacks. At the end of the semester the nutrition students analyzed their diets again. Jessica was happy to see a huge change in her analysis—especially a much lower value for added sugars.

Analysis

Changing eating behaviors is not easy, and understanding food labels is only one part of a much larger picture. Eating habits develop for many reasons and, for many reasons, are difficult to change. People eat not only in response to hunger, but to enjoy food with family and friends, to relieve boredom, to soothe jangled nerves, and just for fun. Foods high in sugar, salt, and fat taste good to most people. Family and cultural influences exert strong effects on a person's eating behavior. For young people still eating at home, their families' eating habits play a large role in their food choices.

Jessica's approach to changing her diet incorporates many elements known to enhance the likelihood of behavior change. Recording her diet helped her understand the nutrient composition of her food choices better. Knowledge about health problems can provide powerful motivation for behavior change, so working with her health teacher to learn about type 2 diabetes was a good idea. Helping her mother out by doing the grocery shopping, meal planning, and cooking allowed Jessica to gently steer her own eating and her family's eating in a more healthful direction. Her time in the grocery store comparing food labels increased her knowledge about food products.

Countless experts have noted that trying to develop a healthful lifestyle in the United States is like swimming upstream. Occupations (and being a student) are sedentary, and food too high in sugar, salt, and unhealthy fats is everywhere. Ideally, people would have an easier time making healthful choices. But until major changes occur in most people's food environments, most people, like Jessica, will need to exert extra effort to make healthful food choices.

4. LIVING WITH CELIAC DISEASE

Anna was not diagnosed with celiac disease until she was 18 years old, although she had experienced symptoms related to the disorder for at least 10 years. Looking back, she wondered how her doctors had missed the diagnosis, but then again, her symptoms had come and gone, and she had often felt fine. She had learned to live with her mysterious rashes and bouts of diarrhea. Everyone figured her iron-deficiency anemia was no big deal, since it was so common in teenage girls. But she saw a new health care provider at the clinic for her pre-college physical who put two and two together. After Anna's blood tests revealed high levels of the antibodies associated with celiac disease, Anna underwent an endoscopy that confirmed the diagnosis.

The relief Anna experienced at finally receiving a diagnosis quickly melted away as she began to confront the difficulties of her dietary restrictions. Anna's provider counseled Anna to avoid all gluten and gave her a pamphlet explaining celiac disease and what foods to avoid. Anna still lived at home with her parents and three younger siblings, where her parents did the grocery shopping and cooking. Both parents worked full time, and Anna felt bad asking them to change the shopping and eating habits for everyone in the house just because Anna had to avoid gluten. She gave them the list of foods she needed to avoid, but with the frequent appearance of pasta at dinner, she could see she was on her own. Anna felt pretty overwhelmed, with her summer waitressing job and getting ready to head off to college.

Anna studied the food labels of every packaged food that entered the house, looking at the allergen statements and ingredients. So many additives and words she had never seen before! She double-checked the ingredient lists against the food list her provider had given her. But the list contained dozens of ingredients. How would she ever be able to avoid them all? She realized that just avoiding the main items, like bread, pasta, breakfast cereals, and pastries, would not get rid of all the gluten in her family's diet. Her parents were well intentioned, buying her special gluten-free bread and cookies. But Anna realized there could still be gluten in the many sauces and condiments regularly used in cooking.

Anna hoped moving to college might solve some of the family meal issues, as the college promised gluten-free options in the dining hall. Anna's head was spinning from all the orientation events, many served up with snacks such as cookies and pizza. Focused on making new friends and figuring out what classes to take, Anna often succumbed to hunger and ate whatever was on hand. Of course, her symptoms came back with a vengeance, and she vowed to be more careful. She began selecting more foods from the gluten-free station in the dining hall, and met some other students with celiac disease, who introduced her to the people running the gluten-free station. But her favorite station was the salad bar. She knew vegetables and fruits were naturally gluten-free and loved heaping her plate with the wonderful produce.

After a few weeks, the school work began to pile up, and Anna found herself fighting fatigue, falling asleep in class and having difficulty focusing on her homework, even though she was getting eight hours of sleep most nights. Worried that her iron-deficiency anemia was getting worse, she visited the health center, where a nurse confirmed her suspicions. The nurse also noted that Anna had lost 5 lbs in the past month, since her pre-college physical. Anna explained her difficulty adjusted to a gluten-free diet, and the nurse gave her a referral to a dietician.

The dietician immediately got Anna back on iron supplements and helped Anna create meal plans that were high in iron but gluten-free. The dietician helped Anna better understand issues of cross-contamination that can occur in a kitchen. Anna could not eat a sandwich, even with gluten-free bread, if it was prepared on a surface that also was used for regular bread. To really eliminate cross-contamination, pots, pans, knives, and other kitchen utensils should be clean, and not recently used for gluten-containing foods. Toasters needed to be dedicated to gluten-free products only. The dietician helped Anna learn to carry gluten-free snacks with her, so that she did not give into the temptation of grabbing a slice of pizza "just this once." At the grocery store, Anna looked for "gluten-free" certifications on food labels, rather than relying only on the ingredient list to avoid gluten-containing ingredients.

Analysis

Many people do not realize what a serious disorder celiac disease is, and how disruptive the diagnosis can be. Eating gluten-free food is especially difficult for young people who do not do their own shopping and cooking. Institutional dining—school cafeterias and college dining halls—can be tricky to navigate, although many are quite careful about offering gluten-free options. Some restaurants are better than others about offering truly gluten-free menu options. Young people with celiac disease often find themselves in social situations featuring gluten-containing foods, such as birthday cakes and pizza. It may take an enormous amount of will power to say no to favorite foods. In addition, many newly diagnosed young people feel awkward eating differently from their friends and peers.

Eating gluten-free becomes easier with time, as people develop new eating behaviors and find new favorite foods. Food labels are indispensable for anyone trying to avoid gluten. While the ingredient list is very helpful, it is not enough, as Anna's story shows. Cross-contamination may allow gluten into products typically made without gluten-containing ingredients. Therefore, people with celiac disease must look for foods that are naturally gluten-free, such as fruits, vegetables, and meats, when they are in the supermarket and cooking at home. They should also rely on gluten-free certifications when purchasing labeled food products to be sure cross-contamination has not occurred.

5. FOOD LABELS AND FARMING: THE BIG PICTURE

Jackson's interest in organic farming started when his friend Sam talked him into WWOOFing during their gap year after high school and before starting college. "Woofing?" Jackson asked. Sam explained that it stood for World Wide Opportunities on Organic Farms. "My cousin did this last year. You work 4–6 hours a day on a farm, and they give you your meals and a place to stay. If you don't mind the work, it's a great way to travel! There are participating farms all over the world. What countries do you want to see?"

Jackson had been saving his money for several months to do some traveling during his gap year, and this sounded perfect. "What about starting in Scandinavia during the summer we graduate, and working our way south as the weather gets colder? We could work in several different counties. We could even go to Africa!"

Living and working on farms for a year made Jackson realize how complicated, difficult, and rewarding farming could be. Growing vegetables was kind of like a miracle—little seeds sending forth sprouts that turned into food. He loved working with the animals, especially on the farms where milk from goats or sheep was made into cheese. Jackson and Sam learned a lot talking to the farm owners, farm workers, and the other WWOOFers they met during their travels.

When his first year of college began, Jackson signed up for a course on agriculture and the environment. Jackson was in his element as the class explored farming practices around the world, and their impact on the environment. The professor challenged the students to look at their own shopping and eating habits to analyze what farming practices they were supporting with their food dollars.

Jackson began reading the labels of the food he purchased more carefully. What did the word "organic" on a food label actually mean? And which cage-free label was the best? Or were they all the same? Each had a website that explained what farming practices were allowed and how farms were (or weren't) inspected.

The biggest variations in label meanings were on the animal products—eggs, dairy, and meat. Jackson had found that European farmers did not have much respect for many agricultural and food production practices in the United States. Jackson had been impressed with animal husbandry practices that he had observed on the small, organic European farms where he had worked. The animals were generally treated pretty well, even the ones being raised for meat. When he had asked one of the farmers how they could kill animals they had raised, the farmer replied, "We treat them well, then they have one bad day."

Jackson created a portfolio of food labels from animal products for one of his class projects. Some of the labels were like a story book. One label from a carton of organic eggs took him several minutes to read thoroughly. There were pictures of the farmers and their families holding the chickens, a verification symbol that read "Certified Humane, Raised and Handled," a statement that the eggs had omega-3 fatty acids, instructions for cooking the eggs to prevent food poisoning, and notes on the recycled packaging. A package of chicken thighs claimed to support local farmers, with Internet links to content explaining more about their business model. Which of these claims and statements was regulated and how? Jackson spent hours on the Internet tracking each one down and exploring the different companies producing the labeled products.

The professor of the agriculture and the environment course included an interesting section on food justice, which Jackson had thought about a lot. How do food systems relate to the social systems in which they operate? How can shoppers select products that support community activities to grow, sell, and eat healthy food? The class had speakers from the local Food Bank Farm and other groups working to increase food security for low-income people in the area.

Jackson also wondered about how people's purchasing habits influence the farming practices of growers near and far. The class looked at coffee growing and learned about the Fair Trade certifications. Jackson learned that the Fair Trade Certified seal indicates that a single ingredient product, like coffee, was produced according to Fair Trade USA's standards. These standards help to make sure that farm workers are fairly paid and work in safe conditions. Farmers of the product are supposed to farm in ways that protect the environment.

The course and Jackson's WWOOFing experience opened Jackson's eyes to the many issues involved in the simple act of shopping for groceries. He knew the aisles of a supermarket would never again look the same.

Analysis

In reality, a food label can never tell consumers everything they might wish to know about a food. Food manufacturers want to put a positive spin on their product and create packaging and label information that makes their product attractive to buyers. The appearance of the USDA Organic program and third-party verifications for farming and animal husbandry methods testify to the presence of consumer interest in purchasing products grown or raised with certain farming practices. These verifications can help provide information to consumers interested in the impact of food production on the environment, the treatment of farm workers, and the animal husbandry practices of farmers providing a given product.

As consumers like Jackson dig more deeply into the meaning of claims and verification emblems on a food label, the labels may generate more questions than answers. Many products have Internet links. Verification seals and label claims have explanatory links as well. Some grocery stores offer information about their suppliers. Food co-ops often research their suppliers carefully to make sure they are supporting groups they approve of.

Some consumers enjoy shopping at local farmers markets. Even though labeling is usually not required on these food products, information can be gathered by talking directly to the farmers producing the food they are selling. Visiting and buying from local farmers and food producers helps to support local economies.

Glossary

Acceptable Macronutrient Distribution Range (AMDR): Recommendations from the Food and Nutrition Board regarding healthful intakes of fat, protein, and carbohydrate.

Allergens: Allergens are substances that cause an allergic response in susceptible people, a type of immune response that, in some cases, can lead to life-threatening symptoms, a condition known as anaphylaxis.

American Academy of Pediatrics (AAP): The leading professional association of pediatricians. The AAP periodically issues guidelines for caretakers regarding good practices in infant and child care.

American Cancer Society (ACS): A nonprofit organization that funds cancer research and educational programs.

American Heart Association (AHA): A nonprofit organization that funds cardiovascular medical research and educates consumers on the prevention of cardiovascular disease.

Calcium: Calcium is the most abundant mineral found in the human body and plays a key role in a variety of functions. It is best known for its importance in the structures of bones and teeth.

Calorie: Calories are a measure of the energy contained in food. Scientists define a calorie as the amount of energy needed to raise the temperature of 1 g of water by 1°C under standard conditions. The calories on food labels are actually kilocalories. One kilocalorie equals 1,000 calories, or the amount of heat needed to raise the temperature of 1 kg of water by 1°C.

Carbohydrates: Carbohydrates are a large group of organic molecules that include sugars, starches, and most types of dietary fiber. Informally, the term "carbohydrate" (or even "carbs") is used to refer to foods that contain relatively high concentrations of carbohydrate molecules.

Celiac disease: A condition in which gluten elicits an autoimmune response, in which immune cells mistakenly attack the lining of the small intestine.

Center for Food Safety and Applied Nutrition (CFSAN): The branch of the FDA that regulates food labeling. Its mission is to be sure the foods people eat in the United States are safe, wholesome, sanitary, and properly labeled, working to ensure that labels are truthful and not misleading.

Centers for Disease Control and Prevention (CDC): A federal agency that conducts and supports health promotion, prevention, and preparedness activities in the United States in order to improve public health.

Cholesterol: Cholesterol belongs to a group of chemical compounds called sterols. Cholesterol is found both in foods and in the body. Cholesterol performs many important functions in the body.

Consumers Union: An independent nonprofit organization, with no financial ties to food producers, governmental organizations such as the FDA or USDA, or to the third-party organizations.

Daily Values: A set of dietary standards used on food labels to help consumers understand the nutrient content of food products. The percent (%) Daily Value tells consumers what percentage of a Daily Value is supplied by one serving of the labeled food product.

Department of Health and Human Services (HHS): A large federal agency charged with enhancing and protecting the health of people in the United States. Its work is done through a variety of divisions, including the Food and Drug Administration (FDA), the Centers for Disease Control and Prevention (CDC), and the National Institutes of Health (NIH).

Dietary fiber: The components of food that cannot be digested in the stomach or small intestine of human beings. Once dietary fiber passes into the large intestine, it influences the nature of the material that eventually forms the stools and interacts with the microorganisms that live in the lower portion of the GI tract.

Dietary Guidelines for Americans: A public health document produced by the USDA that provides an overview and description of guidelines for a healthy diet. Updated every five years, the Dietary Guidelines for Americans helps guide FDA and USDA food labeling, as well as many other important initiatives.

Dietary Reference Intakes (DRI): DRI is the general term for a set of nutrient reference values used to plan and assess nutrient intakes of healthy people. They are developed and published by the Food and Nutrition Board of the Health and Medicine Division of the National Academies of Sciences, Engineering, and Medicine.

Fat: In food, fat is one of the three macronutrients used by the body to make energy. Fat refers to both oils and solid fats in the diet. Oils are liquid at room temperature, while solid fats, like butter or the fat in meat, are solid. On the food label, total fat represents the fat content, including all types of fats, in a serving of a food product.

Federal Register: The daily record of the federal government. It is published each business day by the National Archives and Records Administration's Office of the Federal Register. The *Federal Register* records federal agency actions, including creation of regulations; proposed rules and notices of interest to the public; and executive orders, proclamations, and other documents.

Federal Trade Commission (FTC): A federal agency, the mission of the FTC is to protect consumers by stopping unfair, deceptive, or fraudulent practices in the marketplace. It investigates companies when consumers or agencies like the FDA file complaints.

Food and Drug Administration (FDA): A federal agency, part of the U.S. Department of Health and Human Services. The FDA is charged with protecting public health through the oversight of food; beverages (excluding alcohol); tobacco; cosmetics; human and veterinary drugs; medical devices; biological products, such as vaccines, blood, and tissue; and products that emit radiation, such as ultraviolet lights for tanning and medical imaging devices.

Food and Nutrition Board: A division of the Health and Medicine Division (HMD) of the National Academies of Sciences, Engineering, and Medicine. The Food and Nutrition Board creates the tables of recommended intake level for a variety of nutrients for 22 different population groups, based on age and sex, and, for women, conditions of pregnancy and lactation.

Food intolerances: Distinct from true food allergies, food intolerance symptoms are generally less severe and include intestinal gas, abdominal discomfort, diarrhea, hives, headaches, or irritability and usually come on gradually. These symptoms may result from an absence of an enzyme needed to fully digest a food, irritable bowel syndrome, sensitivity to food additives, reoccurring stress, or psychological factors.

Gluten: A protein found in certain grains, including wheat, rye, and barley. Gluten is the protein people with celiac disease or gluten intolerance must avoid.

Health claims: Statements regarding the association between specific foods or food components and reduced risk of a particular disease or health problem. These claims are regulated by the FDA primarily to prevent food producers from exaggerating the potential health benefits of their products.

Healthy People: A public health document that sets forth science-based 10-year national goals for improving the health of people in the United States. (Health People 2030 is in development.) This document is produced by a large number of organizations, including the National Institutes of Health (NIH), the Centers for Disease Control and Prevention (CDC), and the USDA.

Hydrogenation: A process used by food product manufacturers to make fatty acids in foods more saturated, and thus more stable at room temperature. This stability gives food products a longer shelf life.

Iron: An essential mineral that performs many important functions in the human body. It is best known as a component of the compounds that carry oxygen in the body, but it has other important functions as well.

MyPlate: A nutrition guide designed by the USDA. The MyPlate guide often appears as a visual depiction of a place setting and a glass, divided into five food groups—fruits, grains, vegetables, and protein on the plate, with dairy in the glass.

National Academies of Sciences, Engineering, and Medicine: The collective national scientific academy of the United States. Scientists serving in the Academies are volunteers, nominated by their peers because of their scientific achievements and recognition. People rely on the National Academies for objective, accurate, and unbiased advice on important issues.

National Academy of Medicine (NAM): A division of the National Academies of Sciences, Engineering, and Medicine. Formerly called the Institute of Medicine (IOM)], the NAM is a nonprofit, nongovernmental organization whose goal is to provide unbiased, authoritative advice on issues relating to health and medicine. Scientists serving on the NAM are volunteers, nominated by their peers because of their scientific achievements and recognition.

National Institutes of Health (NIH): An agency under the umbrella of the Department of Health and Human Services that is responsible for funding and guiding biomedical and public health research.

National Organics Program (NOP): A USDA program that regulates the use of the term "organic" on food labels so that consumers can be assured that the term has meaning, and that food products displaying the term on food labels are made with ingredients, or are themselves foods, produced on farms actually using organic farming methods, as defined by the USDA.

National Research Council: The branch of the National Academies of Sciences, Engineering, and Medicine that researches and writes reports that help to guide national policy and inform the public. For example, the National Research Council's 1989 report, "Diet and Health: Implications for Reducing Chronic Disease Risk," helped to guide the FDA's work on food labels.

Nutrient content claim: Statements regarding the amount of a nutrient in a food product. These claims are regulated by the FDA and the USDA so that all food labels use the same standard; that is, a claim such as "low sodium" has the same meaning on all food labels.

Nutrition Facts panel: Also known as the Nutrition Facts label, this chart is mandatory on a majority of food labels and provides information on the nutritional content of the labeled food product. The format of the Nutrition Facts panel and the rules for its use are regulated by the FDA.

Nutrition Labeling and Education Act (NLEA): A law passed by Congress in 1990, the NLEA required nutrition labeling on all packaged food, and that all health claims on packages be standardized. The standardized and mandatory nutrition information debuted on food labels in 1994.

Organic: On a food label, this word indicates that the food has been produced in accordance with rules established by the USDA's National Organics Program (NOP). With the exception of foods produced on very small farms, only products that have been certified by the NOP may use the word "organic" on food labels in the United States.

Potassium: A mineral critical to many cellular and electrical functions in the human body. In general, potassium plays important roles in helping to regulate the body's acid-base balance, build muscles, synthesize proteins, manage fluid balance, metabolize carbohydrates, and regulate electrical activity of the heart and nerves.

Protein: Proteins are nitrogen-containing organic compounds found in all plants and animals. Protein is found throughout the human body, in structures such as muscle and bone; the immune cells that fight infection; the red blood cells that carry oxygen to all parts of the body; neurochemicals and hormones such as serotonin and epinephrine; and the enzymes that regulate biochemical processes such as digestion and energy production. Proteins are composed of smaller units called amino acids.

Reference Amounts Customarily Consumed (RACC): Serving sizes mandated by the FDA to be used on food labels.

Saturated fats (sat fat): Saturated fats, often abbreviated as "sat fat" on food labels, are a type of fat. Saturated fats refer to fatty acids in which the bonds between carbon atoms are all single. Single carbon-carbon bonds are more stable than double bonds and affect the behavior of these fatty acids.

Serving size: On food labels, serving size reflects portions customarily consumed at one sitting. Values on the Nutrition Facts panel are given per serving size of the food product. Because "serving size" is a rather vague term, the FDA uses the term "Reference Amounts Customarily Consumed" (RACC) in its literature for food manufacturers, and publishes a table for food producers to consult when they are creating labels.

Sodium: An essential nutrient, a mineral found primarily in salts. Table salt is the primary source of sodium in the diet, and the terms "salt" and "sodium" are often used interchangeably when discussing dietary recommendations. Sodium performs many essential functions in the body.

Structure/function claims: Statements that describe possible effects of a food, food component, or dietary supplement component on body structures or functions, such as bone health, digestion, or immune system function. Structure/function claims may say that foods support health, but not make claims that the food can treat or cure a disease. These claims are regulated by the FDA.

Sugars: Also known as simple carbohydrates, sugars are relatively small molecules of carbohydrate found naturally in fruits and vegetables, as well as milk. Sugars are also found in sweeteners that are added to food products.

Tolerable upper intake level (UL): The highest level of a nutrient intake that is likely to pose no risk of adverse health effects for most people. These levels are set by the Food and Nutrition Board of the National Academy of Medicine.

Trans fatty acids (trans fats): A type of fat, usually created by hydrogenation, a process used by food product manufacturers to make fatty acids in foods more saturated, thus more stable and with a longer shelf life. While trans fats technically have a carbon-carbon double bond, the arrangement of other atoms around the bond leads to a shape of the fatty acid that is more similar to saturated fatty acids. Greater intake of trans fats in the diet has been linked to higher rates of artery disease.

United States Department of Agriculture (USDA): A federal department that oversees the U.S. agricultural economy. Its goal is to provide a safe, sufficient, and nutritious food supply for the American people. The USDA represents the interests of farmers and ranchers; promotes agricultural production; administers food assistance programs to low-income people; inspects and regulates labeling of certain food products; and generates healthy diet guidelines and information.

Unsaturated fats: A type of fat, unsaturated fatty acids have at least one carbon-carbon double bond. Monounsaturated fatty acids have one carbon-carbon double bond, while polyunsaturated fatty acids have more than one. The location of this carbon-carbon double bond helps to name the fatty acid and affects the fatty acid's structure and behavior in the body.

U.S. Customs and Border Protection (CBP): A federal agency that enforces certain labeling requirements in accordance with U.S. and international trade regulations. The CBP is a part of the Department of Homeland Security, that is charged with safeguarding U.S. borders to protect the public "from dangerous people and materials while enhancing the Nation's global economic competitiveness by enabling legitimate trade and travel." Some of its rules govern food imported from other countries and sold in the United States.

Vitamin A: a fat-soluble vitamin that facilitates many critical physiological processes in the body. It is best known for its important roles in vision.

Vitamin C: also known as ascorbic acid, is a water-soluble vitamin. Vitamin C's functions include assisting in collagen production, intensifying the body's absorption of iron, aiding in wound healing, and maintaining healthy bones and teeth.

Vitamin D: A fat-soluble vitamin that is converted to a chemical that functions as a hormone in the body. Vitamin D is often referred to as the "sunshine vitamin" as the body can make vitamin D from a precursor in the skin, when the skin is exposed to ultraviolet B radiation from the sun.

World Health Organization (WHO): An agency of the United Nations that is concerned with international public health.

Directory of Resources

RELEVANT ORGANIZATIONS AND WEBSITES

For more information on food label regulations and nutrition, go to the websites of the U.S. Department of Agriculture (USDA) and the U.S. Food and Drug Administration (FDA). Sections of their websites that are especially helpful include the following:

United States Department of Agriculture—Food and Nutrition Information Center. https://www.nal.usda.gov/fnic.

United States Food and Drug Administration—Labeling & Nutrition. https://www.fda.gov/food/labelingnutrition/default.htm

The section of the website most related to food labels is the following:

National Agricultural Library, United States Department of Agriculture (n.d.) General information and resources for food labeling. Retrieved from https://www.nal.usda.gov/fnic/general-information-and-resources-food-labeling

Hundreds of interesting articles written for consumers as well as food manufacturers may be found on the Food section of the FDA website.

U.S. FDA. (Updated regularly). Food. Retrieved from https://www.fda.gov/Food/default.htm

The USDA's choosemyplate.gov website has many good articles on healthy eating, including dietary guidelines, recipes and menus, and eating on a budget:

U.S. Department of Agriculture. (2019). What is MyPlate? Retrieved from https://www.choosemyplate.gov/WhatIsMyPlate

Other organizations with helpful websites include the following. All offer articles on nutrition and food labels.

Academy of Nutrition and Dietetics. https://www.eatright.org/food# Nutrition

American Heart Association—"Eat a Healthy Diet." https://www.heart .org/en/healthy-living/healthy-eating/eat-smart/nutrition-basics

Center for Science in the Public Interest. https://cspinet.org/eating-healthy

ConsumerReports, Greener Choices. http://greenerchoices.org/labels/

Harvard T.H. Chan School of Public Health. https://www.hsph.harvard .edu/nutritionsource/

BOOKS

Readers interested in learning more about nutrition and health will find good information in the following basic nutrition encyclopedia. This work, arranged with entries in alphabetical order, presents comprehensive overviews of over 200 nutrition and health topics, along with suggested readings for each topic.

Brehm, B. A. (Ed.). (2015) *Nutrition: Science, Issues, and Applications.* Santa Barbara, CA: Greenwood Press.

Introductory college nutrition texts often include a chapter on tools for diet design. These tools include not only food labels but also various dietary guidelines and other public health initiatives. The two texts listed next are easy-to-read and comprehensive introductory texts. They are regularly updated, so look for the most recent editions.

Insel, P., Ross, D., McMahon, K., & Bernstein, M. (2018). *Discovering nutrition.* Sudbury, MA: Jones and Bartlett Learning.

Smith, A. M., Collene, A. L., & Spees, C. K. (2019). *Wardlaw's contemporary nutrition.* New York, NY: McGraw-Hill Education.

A book on nutrition labeling by the National Academy of Sciences includes a very readable and interesting chapter on the recent history of food labeling. This book is available online.

Institute of Medicine (US) Committee on Examination of Front-of-Package Nutrition Rating Systems and Symbols; Wartella, E. A.,

Lichtenstein, A. H., & Boon, C.S., (Eds.). (2010). *Front-of-package nutrition rating systems and symbols: Phase 1 report*; Chapter 2. History of nutrition labeling. Washington, D.C.: National Academy of Sciences. Retrieved from https://www.ncbi.nlm.nih.gov/books/NBK209859/

GOVERNMENT RECORDS

Readers really wanting to dig into labeling regulations might find the final rule governing the revision of the Nutrition Facts panel of interest. This 258-page document is well organized and provides not only the labeling rules update but also the rationale for many of the changes.

Food and Drug Administration, Department of Health and Human Services. (2016, May 27). *Food labeling: Revision of the nutrition and supplement facts labels*. Washington, D.C.: *Federal Register*, Government Printing Office. Retrieved from https://www.gpo.gov/fdsys/pkg/FR-2016-05-27/pdf/2016-11867.pdf

The Electronic Code of Federal Regulations (e-CFR) lists the rules published in the *Federal Register* by the executive departments and federal government agencies, including the FDA and the USDA. The e-CFR is updated daily and thus contains the most current list of rulings related to the FDA and USDA.

Electronic Code of Federal Regulations. (Updated daily). Title 21—Food and Drugs; Chapter 1—Food and Drug Administration, Department of Health and Human Services. Retrieved from https://www.ecfr.gov/cgi-bin/text-idx?SID=bfd7401d47b671ad128fa55184c83641&mc=true&tpl=/ecfrbrowse/Title21/21cfr101_main_02.tpl

Index

About the Author

Barbara A. Brehm, EdD, is professor and chair of the Department of Exercise and Sport Studies at Smith College, Northampton, Massachusetts, where she teaches courses on nutrition and health and sports nutrition. Dr. Brehm writes extensively on nutrition; her publications include Greenwood's two-volume *Nutrition: Science, Issues, and Applications*.